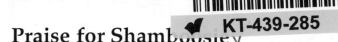

KT-439-285

Praise for Shamboosie

*"In this instructional guide, Shamboosie, **a color master consultant, gives helpful tips and simple techniques for achieving beautiful, healthy hair,** explaining the do's and don'ts, the whys and why nots of proper care."*
—**Ann Burns, Editor,** *Library Journal*

*"**Very informative!** Shamboosie is a legend to the hair industry."*
—**John Blassingame, Publisher,** *Today's Black Woman*

*"**Beautiful Black Hair** is a great guide for all women of color. It tells you what to expect at a salon and teaches you how to care for your hair at home between salon visits. **A must read.**"*
—**Charlene Carroll, Co-Author,**
  ***Milady's Standard System of Salon Skills** and*
  Owner, Charlene's Hair Salon

*"**Every model should own this book!** Beautiful hair is vital in our business and Shamboosie shows us how we can have it all the time."*
—**Dee Simmons Edelstein, Former Director,**
  Grace Del Marco Models

*"Shamboosie has simplified the steps toward having beautiful hair. He has answered so many questions and helped me to understand the best techniques and products for home hair care maintenance. **Read this, and you too can have long, beautiful, healthy hair.**"*
—**Yvonne Rose, Co-Author,** *Is Modeling For You?*
  The Handbook and Guide for the Young Aspiring
  Black Model

Beautiful Black Hair

Real Solutions to Real Problems

By Shamboosie

Amber Books
New York   Los Angeles
Phoenix

Beautiful Black Hair: Real Solutions to Real Problems

by Shamboosie

Published by:
Amber Books
A Division of Amber Communications Group, Inc.
1334 East Chandler Boulevard, Suite 5-D67
Phoenix, AZ 85048
amberbk@aol.com
www.amberbooks.com

Tony Rose, Publisher/Editorial Director
Yvonne Rose, Associate Publisher/Senior Editor
Design

Samuel P. Peabody, Associate Publisher
The Printed Page, Interior & Cover

© Copyright 2002, 2007 by Shamboosie and Amber BOOKS
ISBN 13: 978-0-9702224-6-6 / ISBN 10: 0-9702224-6-7

Library of Congress Cataloging-In-Publication Data
Shamboosie.
    Beautiful black hair : real solutions to real problems / by Shamboosie
        p. cm.
    ISBN 0-9702224-6-7
        1. Hair--Care and hygiene. 2. African-American women--Health and hygiene. 3. Beauty, Personal. I. Title.

RL91.S47 2002
646.7'24--dc21

10 9 8 7 6 5 4 3 2 1

2002018512

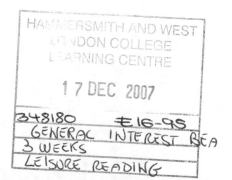

Dedication

To The Beautiful Women of Color in my life:

In memory of my mother, Remaetha
In honor of my stepmother, Mattie
In honor of my wife, Marilyn
In honor of my sisters:
Emma Jean
Marie
Helen
Mavis & Denise

In memory of my sister Margaret

In honor of my daughters:
Angela
Sharon
Brittanie & Deandra

In honor of my granddaughters:
LaQuida
Shamikka
Mashonda
Tashee, Tanika, and Miranda

I Love You All!

Acknowledgments

First I want to thank God for the miracle of this book. I realize He has been with me all my life, and the only way I could have done this is with His love for me, and His help. I trust Him, I love Him, I totally depend on Him, and I owe it all to Him.

My deepest appreciation to my Publisher, Tony Rose, and Amber Books. I thank you from the bottom of my heart for taking a chance on my work. Your advice and direction has helped tremendously.

Special thanks to Yvonne Rose for helping me to articulate my thoughts. We worked well together, and I don't know what I would have done without her expertise.

May God bless both of you many times for believing in me.

Janell Walden Agyeman, Literary Agent: Thanks for believing in me and in this project. I appreciate all of your encouragement, all of your time and efforts on my behalf. You are special! You are an angel.

Wade Hudson, Advisor and friend: Thanks for your encouraging words that started the ball rolling. I appreciate your inspiring words of counsel and your guidance. You took time from your busy schedule to help a newcomer get started. I am very grateful for your introduction to Janell.

Phillda Ragland-Njau, Technical Support: Thanks for everything. You were there every step of the way. You were an invaluable source of inspiration. Thanks for your diligence and hard work. I can never thank you enough.

Hattie Hughes, Mentor: The gift you gave me has enabled to see the world through words—words that have painted the very face of God, His love, His presence, and His being in my heart. I thank you for believing in me. You challenged me to pursue and to persevere. I thank God that you crossed my path. You changed my life!

Thurston Evans, Cosmetology Instructor: I am so grateful you took the time to teach me how to style hair. You taught me the how's, the why's, and to see the finish from the beginning. Most of all, I am grateful that you taught me how to teach others. I thank you from the bottom of my heart.

Marilyn J. Dixon, Technical Support: You are my best friend as well as the love of my life. I thank God for you. We are partners in all things, and I could not have done this without you!

Foreword

Shamboosie is a passionate visionary sharing the proper understanding of hair care by providing real solutions to real problems. Shamboosie is a man blessed by The Creator with the gift of "understandable articulation." I know because he was my teacher of Advanced Training at Dudley Cosmetology University. Later, when I became a teacher, I was privileged to work closely with him as a colleague. I realized early on that when Shamboosie teaches, you always "get it." There's never any confusion because he always makes it clear. Shamboosie's dedication is underscored by his desire to help you develop the confidence to apply the knowledge you attain. With "hairdressing skills to pay the bills," this teacher is one of a kind.

In *Beautiful Black Hair: Real Solutions to Real Problems* laypersons as well as hairstylists will learn the "how's," the "why's" and the "why not's." Among the many application methods, timely tips, and proper hair care techniques, you will learn how to combat the troublesome problems of dryness, breakage, and hair loss. You will learn about hair care products and how to use them correctly. You will learn what hair is made of, how it grows, and how to keep it healthy, and much, much more.

Beautiful Black Hair will teach you practically everything you ever wanted to know about hair but no one was willing to tell you— until now!

Shamboosie keeps the reading "light" by interspersing authentic anecdotes from his life and career that make this book fun to read.

Beautiful Black Hair is "right on time" and "right on target." After reading this book, you will be motivated and well- equipped to make the commitment to do what is right for your hair.

Beautiful Black Hair is instructional as well as enjoyable, and it is written in a simple, easy to follow style. A smile will light your face when you realize that you have discovered many secrets that you never knew about hair care.

Beautiful Black Hair really does live up to its promise to furnish real solutions to real problems. This is the one we've all been waiting for! Enjoy!

> Frederick Parnell
> The Primp Club
> Image Hair Service
> Brooklyn, NY

Contents

Introduction

A woman's hair should be her crowning glory. If it is not, she may desire it to be so. This is a sentiment shared by women all over the world. When a woman's hair looks good, she feels good, her self-esteem soars, and she is ready to face the world. Every woman can have beautiful hair.

It is my prayer that this book will teach you to take good care of your hair, to love your hair, and to enjoy doing what it takes to insure the beauty of your hair. It is my sincere wish, as a black man and as a hair care professional, to help the black woman to attain and maintain along with her natural good looks, beautiful healthy hair.

The Black woman, however, has become confused and frustrated in her search for a glowing crown of beautiful hair. The Black woman does so many things to her hair-she cuts it, perms it, relaxes it, colors it, and weaves it. Innocent mistakes, such as misuse of hair care products and over-processing have caused severe chemical damage in the form of dullness, extreme dryness, and hair loss. When she realizes that something has gone wrong, she doesn't know exactly what to do or where to turn for help.

Beautiful Black Hair is written to give you the real answers to your real hair care problems. It is my hope that this book will be viewed as the standard solutions textbook of cosmetology for today's women of color. In this book you will get the truth, the whole truth, and nothing but the truth. This is my pledge and my promise to you.

Beautiful Black Hair: Real Solutions to Real Problems is the conclusive hair care handbook that will take the mystery out of Black hair care. This instructional guide contains helpful tips and simple techniques for achieving beautiful healthy hair, and answers the questions that have puzzled so many for so long. This book explains the do's and don'ts and the why's and why not's of proper hair care in a clear, easy-to-understand format.

Beautiful Black Hair is unique in its scope and content. In addition to providing real solutions to real hair care problems, I will share authentic stories from my personal and professional life.

This is the first black hair care book to:

- ❑ Outline daily maintenance regimens in easy-to-follow steps
- ❑ Address hair care problems for all types of hair
- ❑ Dispel the myths associated with black hair care
- ❑ Tackle the tough hair care questions with honesty and clarity.

Two of the most important topics discussed are: Relaxers-Lye and No-Lye, and the proper use of Conditioners.

Not all women wear chemical relaxers, but for those that do, I will explain the "no burn technique." This is an application technique that guarantees no scalp burns when the proper method is utilized.

Understanding of the basics is vital to understanding proper hair care, and you will learn what hair is, beginning with the three layers of the hair, the cuticle, the cortex, and the medulla.

You will also learn the key to hair growth and the answer to the most common hair growth questions.

Hair breakage is a very serious problem that many women experience, and Beautiful Black Hair provides the answers that will stop breakage and end dry brittle hair forever.

Hair color has risen in popularity and this often misunderstood subject is explained in an easy-to- follow, step-by-step method.

Recognizing diversity in style and preference, a chapter on Natural Hair Care and alternatives such as extensions, weaves, and wigs is included.

The importance of purchasing products especially designed to treat the circumstances of one's hair is stressed. When the proper hair care products are used correctly, the desired results will occur.

You will learn what certain types of hair care products are designed to do, when they should be used, and why.

Caring for children's hair can be a challenging task, whether at home or in the salon. I will share my personal and professional experiences, along with recommendations to help mothers, in an entire chapter that addresses children's hair care solutions.

Beautiful Black Hair has something for everyone—mothers seeking advice for the care of children's hair; teenagers experimenting with the latest trends and styles; college students in need of quick and easy hair management; business women desiring a professional look to fit a busy lifestyle; as well as older women looking for low maintenance help for their hair.

Beautiful Black Hair: Real Solutions to Real Problems is the one that women have been waiting for!

It is my prayer that this book will help you to love and enjoy taking care of your hair at home and enjoy your visits to the salon. God bless you.

Shamboosie

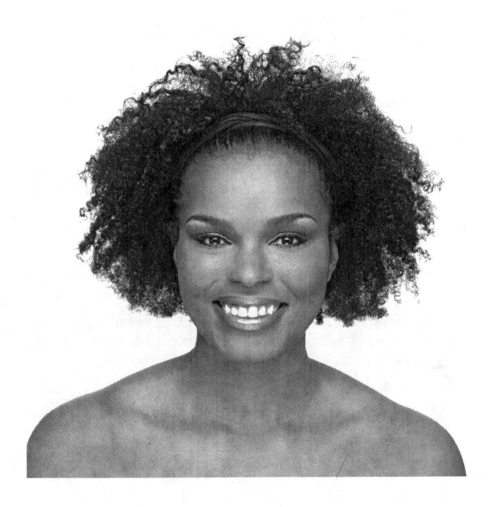

Chapter One

Hair Basics

Hair—What Is It?

Hair is a slender, thin, thread-like fiber composed mostly of pro-tein, also referred to as *keratin*. Hair can be found all over the body, most noticeably growing on the scalp, arm pits and other secret places. There are possibly hundreds of thousands of hair strands growing all over the body.

Trichology, the study of hair, concerns itself with the *papilla, bulb, follicle, root,* and the hair *shaft.* The root of the hair is located beneath the surface of the skin. Wrapped around the root is the hair follicle, a kind of cavity out of which the hair shaft begins, grows, and extends above the surface of the skin and scalp, like that of a beautiful rose.

Then there is the papilla, located at the bottom most portion of the hair shaft and inside the bulb, which is rounded and tear-shaped.

The bottom end of the appendage or hair strand is where the hair receives its nourishment. The size and shape of the hair is deter-mined by the size and shape of the follicle. If the opening of the fol-licle is round, the hair will be straight. If the follicle is flat, the hair will be curly or kinky, the kind of hair many women of color have. If the follicle is oval-shaped, the hair will be wavy. There are some people of color who have all three types and shapes.

1

The Three Layers—Cuticle, Cortex, and Medulla

The first layer of the hair is *the cuticle* or the protective layer. When magnified a thousand times, the cuticle looks like the scales on the back of a fish. When chemicals are applied to the hair shaft, they raise the cuticles allowing product access into the second layer of the hair, the cortex.

The healthier the cuticle layer of the hair is, the healthier the hair will be, and the longer it will grow. The problem women of color have is that they are doing many of the wrong things to the hair, which causes their hair to fall out before the time of its normal cycle.

Hair grows about one-half inch per month. Normally, you will shed an average of about fifty strands per day. Don't let that frighten you. The pieces could be full strands, but in most cases, they are very small pieces of different sizes. At the same time all of this is taking place, the hair is still growing.

I always tell my clients that if they didn't follow the advice I give them for healthy hair, they will end up looking just like me. You see, I shave my head, and I am completely bald. Very few women desire that look, I am sure. Most do not want to look like Shamboosie.

The length that the hair will grow varies with the race, sex and age of the person. Women normally grow hair faster than men. If one does the right things to care for and keep the hair healthy, there is no reason why most people cannot grow a full, long, beautiful head of hair.

It is important to remember that once hair grows out of the scalp, it has no life of its own. It has no way to regenerate itself, so you or a well-trained hair stylist must care for it. The outer layer, the cuticle, must be protected. The key here is to use the right conditioners.

The cortex, or the second layer, is where everything you put on or into your hair, enters through the cuticles. This includes shampoos, conditioners, haircolor, chemicals and even water. The cortex is where the bonds are located, and where peroxide-based haircolors, relaxers, curl perms, conditioners and other chemicals will cause a more permanent change in the hair texture, pigmentation and wave pattern. The bonds of the hair will be discussed later on. The biggest changes occur in the hair from the inside out, and many of those changes are permanent.

A very well-conditioned cuticle layer protects the cortex. When the cuticle is badly damaged, the cortex is exposed. The hair becomes weak, lifeless, and almost impossible to manage. If left this way for too long, which is the case most often, the hair will fall out.

The Medulla, the third layer, is the one that we will not spend much time talking about, because most black hair does not have a medulla. One or more can be found in other hair types, however. The more medullas, the softer and more porous the hair will be. The term porous means the hair's ability to absorb moisture.

 An Awareness Tip: Haircolor, bleach, and thio, also known as the curly perm, all will cause the three layers to become very soft and porous, especially the cuticle. The chemical relaxer also causes soft-ness, but not as much as the others. Depending on the degree of alteration, repair may be possible. The repair, however, will be temporary with little damage, and not possible at all, if the damage is severe. In every case, use a very good protein, mois-turizing conditioner, with emphasis on protein. Only the best will do.

Anytime chemicals are misused, the chance of hair loss is almost 100 percent guaranteed. The chance of saving the hair is slim, but it is possible. Keep in mind that once these chemicals are put in the hair, the changes they make in the structure and texture of the hair are chemical changes, and these changes cannot be reversed.

A Very Surprising Note

With the exception of the conditioning Lye relaxer, the application of every other chemical, including permanent haircolor, curly perms (the curl) and bleach, or a mixture of all four, will cause the hair shaft to become weaker with time. The only exception is hair that is very well cared for or very well conditioned. Everything else will become more damaged and more difficult to manage as time passes. This is the reason why learning about your hair is so important.

1. You must know exactly what you are doing to your hair at all times and just as important, why you are doing it.

2. You should also know what the outcome will be and its affect on your hair before you do things to your hair.

Hair Care Products: The Good, The Bad and The Ugly

There are many different product categories, and they differ depending upon where they are purchased. Beauty salons will usually feature the very best hair care products, if they are products that can only be purchased in a salon.

Whenever I start to work with new clients, I will ask them to bring all of the **Hair Care Products** they have at home with them on their next visit to the salon, so that I can see what they have been using on their hair. Usually, I will look the products over, and get rid of most of them. Then I will give them a list of all the right products to purchase before leaving the salon. Most people will use all of the wrong things, and much of what they have been using has done more harm than good. I prescribe a complete new line up of **Hair Care Products** that cover every area that deals with their individual hair type. I tell them what each product is for, exactly how it should be used, how much, when, and how often each product should be used.

Many of the leading companies have made their complete product line available exclusively to the hair care professional. Consumers may purchase these products in the salon. Actually this is in the client's best interest because the hairstylist, who is familiar with the client's hair, should be able to advise clients as to what products are best suited for their hair structure and overall condition. You and your stylist should always use the same line of **Hair Care Products.** You can also find many of the top **Hair Care Products** in major beauty supply chain stores. The local privately owned beauty supply store, however, usually features an array of low-end **Hair Care Products.**

There are also **Hair Care Products** that are sold in retail establishments such as drug stores, food markets, and department store chains. Here is where the biggest difference in **Hair Care Products** for black hair is found. These types of establishments display black **Hair Care Products** in a little section, a shelf or two, where you will find the worse, most out-dated products on display.

It seems that the buyers for these stores have absolutely no clue as to what is currently going on in the area of ethnic hair care. Therefore, they continue to supply their stores with **Hair Care Products** that are out of date and out of touch with current trends. Remember this, if it comes in a kit, many times it's not fit for your hair, especially the *No-Lye Relaxer.*

So What Is A Woman To Do?

The area of **Hair Care Products** is one that is very often ignored and not addressed in most salons. You must insist on knowing everything about the **Hair Care Products** used on your hair and not just focusing on the finished look. For healthy hair, it is necessary that you understand how best to use products for the maximum affect on your hair for maintenance at home.

The Proof Is In The Pudding

As part of the Cosmetic Arts and Science Industry for more than twenty years, I have come to recognize the difficulty that black mothers, and black women in general, experience when trying to care for their hair and the hair of their daughters.

A very large portion of the black females in the country, are wearing weaves, braids, extensions and wigs because they have lost so much hair from using *No-Lye Relaxer.*

Case in point, I was talking with Mavis Regina, my kid sister, about putting home relaxer kits in her own hair. I told her, that *No-Lye*

Relaxer is no good for the hair. To my surprise she said, " I can't find a **Conditioning Lye Relaxer Kit** that has everything I need in it to do my relaxer." She was speaking of the relaxer, neutralizing shampoo, conditioner, gloves and such. She went on to say "I have to buy everything in separate containers and many of them in larger sizes than I need." If this sounds like I have been spying on you, then chances are your hair is in the same condition as Mavis Regina's.

 A Note of Interest

> Buying your **Hair Care Products** in separate containers is the best way because it allows you to get the highest quality with every item and the exact ones for your hair. If you buy in large quantities it is okay because you will eventually use it up and have to buy more anyway. So stop your fussing and get on with it.

It's A Family Affair

Hair Care Products should be selected depending on the condition and needs of your hair. Whether you are using relaxers, permanent haircolor, doing roller sets, shampoo blow-dry and curl, dandruff treatments or other services, there is a Care Package Prescription that will meet your needs. It is always best to purchase and use products in the *same* brand name family because they are designed to work together, and they contain many of the same ingredients. Each product in the line compliments the next. It's a family affair.

I send every client home with some kind of a **Hair Care Package.** I keep track of it, and replenish it when it runs out. I use only the very best **Hair Care Products**, and insist that my clients use the same line of products, for home maintenance, that I use in the salon. You should insist also. My clients must use the same **Hair Care Products** I use or I will refuse to service their hair. The reason is both consequential and in their favor. It ensures the best possible results for the healthiest hair. It is also the only way I can deliver on my promise to provide the best care possible for their hair. Follow my lead and you can't go wrong.

Awareness Tip:
Whenever you buy any **Hair Care Product,** including the product you have been using for a while, read every word on the label, front and back before using the product on your hair. Pay close attention to all of the warnings, the do's and don'ts, and follow the directions precisely. When you build new habits for taking care of your hair, your hair will build new habits of hanging around much *"longer."*

Generic-The Price is Right

It is a fact that higher quality products mean higher prices. I recommend that if you can afford to do so, buy name brand **Hair Care Products.** Purchasing conditioners and shampoos in smaller sizes may lower the cost. However, if necessary, you can use a generic brand.

Generic hair care products were created when a group of chemists with a long history of making quality **Hair Care Products** decided they could make products as good as the name brands. They could sell them for a lot less, and with the right marketing strategy, they could attract buyers to purchase these products. It worked.

Perhaps generic is the right way for you to go. So how do you know which products are right for you, and how do you know if they are as good as the brand names? Get a name brand product and compare it with a generic brand. The ingredients should read about the same.

I have included a partial list solely for the purpose of helping you make the best selections. It is not important to know what these terms mean or how they work in the products, how they work in your hair, or even how to pronounce them. That is a job for the chemist and not for you or me. Keep in mind that the top brands and best **Hair Care Products** on the market are made with the highest quality of raw materials available, which is why they are the best.

It is not the brand name that makes a **Hair Care Product** a high quality product, it is the quality of raw materials used to make the product. Many of the generic brands are also high quality. These are some of the main ingredients:

▼ Rosemary Extract
▼ Spearmint Oil
▼ Jojoba Oil
▼ Cetyl Alcohol
▼ Keratin Amino Acids
▼ Chamomile Extract
▼ Panthenol
▼ Citric Acid
▼ Potassium Choride
▼ Hydrolyed Keratin
▼ Kelp Extract
▼ Steapyrium Chloride
▼ Stearalkonium
▼ Hanna Extract
▼ Stearyl Alcohol
▼ Fragrance
▼ Propylparaben
▼ Quaternium 15
▼ Deionized Water
▼ Quaternium 48
▼ Steareth 2
▼ Aloe Vera Gel
▼ FD&C Blue No.1
▼ Methylchloroisothiazolinone and
▼ Methylisothiazlinone

Always Remember...

A true professional should be able to tell you everything you need to know about your hair.

I can tell:

❑ If you are wearing a wig, I can tell.

❑ If you are wearing a weave, I can tell.

❑ If you have no-lye relaxer in your hair, I can tell.

❑ If there is a lye relaxer in your hair, I can tell.

❑ If there is both curl and relaxer in your hair, I can tell.

❑ If you put in your own relaxer retouch, I can tell.

❑ If you have permanent haircolor in your hair, and even if the shade is identical to your natural haircolor, I can tell.

❑ If there is bleach in your hair, and even if you have toned it to your own natural haircolor, I can tell.

❑ If your hair is severely damaged, I can tell.

❑ The length of time since your last relaxer, I can tell.

❑ If your hair is coming out by the hand full, I can tell.

❑ If you have been using cheap hair care products, I can tell.

❑ If someone has done something to damage your hair, I can tell.

❑ If there is a curl in your hair, and someone tried to chemically relax the hair, I can tell.

❑ If you haven't shampooed and conditioned your hair in weeks or months, I can tell.

❑ If you have been combing relaxer through your hair, I can tell.

❑ If you are using the wrong kinds of oils in your hair and if you are using them the wrong way, I can tell.

❑ If you have allowed bleach to remain in your hair too long, I can tell.

❑ If the wrong volume of developer was used while putting color in your hair, I can tell.

❑ If you have been given a lousy haircut, I can tell

❑ If it is possible for you to grow a full, long, healthy head of hair, I can tell.

❑ What are the best choices of hair care product for your hair, I can tell.

❑ What is the best kind of relaxer for your hair, I can tell.

❑ What are the best shampoos and conditioners for your hair, I can tell.

❑ If you have any other questions you need answers to concerning your hair, and your family's hair, go on-line and type in the keyword—Shamboosie or E-mail shamboosie@aol.com, I can tell.

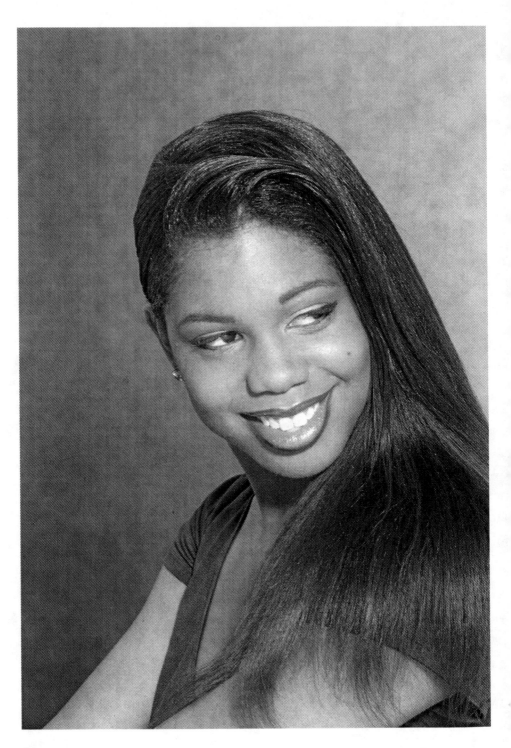

Chapter Two

It's Growing: Understanding Hair Growth

A Conditioning Basic—the Truth and Nothing but the Truth!

The hair shaft is composed of three layers. The first layer is called the *cuticle* or the protective layer. This is also the most important layer. The better you take care of this layer of your hair, the stronger it will be, and the longer your hair will grow. I have always told my clients that the secret to growing their hair is *keeping it on the head*. The answer is found in the theory of "Less is More." The less you do that damages your hair, and the better you care for it, the more beautiful your hair will be.

I don't mean you shouldn't get a haircut, have your ends trimmed, or wear your hair very short, if you choose. However, if it is your desire to have longer healthier hair, you must *stop* doing those things that cause your hair to fall out. Some examples are:

❑ The improper use of permanent haircolor and developers

❑ The use and the improper use of home relaxer kits such as the No-Lye Relaxer

❑ The use of facial soap or dishwashing liquid instead of a pH-balanced shampoo

❑ The use of cheap shampoos and conditioners, which is just like not using a shampoo and conditioner at all.

Some people *never* use conditioners. Others use conditioners, but not on a regular basis. There are even those who are of the opinion that shampooing and conditioning once a month, every ninety days, or even once every six months is sufficient. This may be hard to believe, but the only time some people's hair comes in contact with water, is when they go swimming, get caught in the rain, or when they attempt to do chemical services at home. That is sad, very sad, but true.

Let It Rest, Please! Let It Rest

Some of you have done so many different things to your hair— permed it, bleached it, wrapped and tapped it, braided it, weaved it, "fried it" and dyed it. Maybe it's time to give the hair a break and just "let it rest." Actually, giving your hair a break is a good idea, but not keeping it clean and well-conditioned won't help one bit. There are many things you *should stop* doing, but shampooing and conditioning with very good **Hair Care Products** is essential. So please don't include shampooing and conditioning on your *"things to take a break from"* list.

You should stop doing your own haircoloring and bleaching, and you should definitely stop using home relaxer kits. You should have never started doing those things to your hair in the first place. There is so much that you must be aware of concerning the products you've been putting in your hair. Those things you didn't know are the things that have been causing most of your hair problems.

Take Three Pills and Call Me in a Week

If I were to give you a pill and tell you it would make your hair grow, would you take the pill, even if you had no information to verify my claims? Taking such a pill would be the same as putting chemicals in your hair and not knowing the outcome before hand. The pill could do irreparable damage to your body.

Likewise, your hair can suffer irreparable damage if you are not aware of what is being done *to it* and used *on it*.

A Growing Tip: Remember, once the hair grows out of the scalp, it has no life of it's own, no nerve endings, no way to repair itself. The only way your hair can react to neglect is by becoming difficult to manage and turning a weird color. After a period of time, the hair simply "gives up" on you feeding and taking care of it regularly. The result of such neglect is that the hair falls off your head altogether. Your hair must be taken care of either by you or by a well-trained hair care professional, if you expect to have lovely hair. The way to do this is by shampooing and conditioning very often with the best product money can buy. Remember, you must protect the outer layer, the cuticle.

It's Growing

Whether you realize it of not, your hair is constantly growing. The black woman has long had to deal with scalp pain while trying to comb and style hair that is tightly curled or kinky. I realize most women don't like the way kinky hair looks around the face and hairline, especially when the rest of her hair has been relaxed. The only time she gets any relief from the scalp pain is when she gets her hair retouched or relaxed.

The term "retouch" is synonymous with the term "new growth," which means, *newly grown* hair. This refers to hair you did not have just a few weeks earlier. If you were to get a "new growth retouch" on schedule every six to eight weeks, you would have your hair retouched eight or nine times each year. Remember, your hair is growing all the time. It grows a quarter to one-half inch per month, which is about six inches a year.

It's Growing. Like everything else in your life, your hair has a natural cycle or life span. The growth cycle is different for everyone. Your hair will never last forever, but hair can and will grow long for most humans. Just *keep it on the head* because It's Growing.

An Imperative Scenario

To focus on the importance of caring for the cuticle layer of the hair, I want to emphasize the phrase "**It's Growing.**" Have you ever noticed that most of the things we purchase that are of real value come to us in protective packaging, such as TV's, medication, VCR's, computers, pantyhose, even eggs, and other foods. Strong and secure outer packaging is required to protect these items because they are handled many times before reaching the consumer. The same can be said about hair. This should sound a bit like your hair. Does it?

It's Growing. The cuticle, or outer layer of the hair, is the packaging which protects the valuable content of your hair. The cortex and the medulla, the second and third layers. It is important to take the best care of your hair's protective packaging, which is the cuticle. Your hair will normally need conditioning every three to five days, in addition to a deep conditioning treatment with a concentrated product, every four weeks and after every chemical service.

 A Growing Tip:
When combing wet hair, spray in some conditioning setting lotion, even if you are going to blow the hair dry and hot curl it. Use a large tooth comb to detangle your hair. The conditioning setting lotion will soften the cuticles and allow easier combing. Always begin combing in small sections, at the ends of the hair, and continue combing to the scalp, when detangling.

Under Lock and Key

It's Growing. Your desire and ability to care for your hair properly is the key that will unlock the opportunities for wonderful healthy hair. I use the term "unlock" because making the time to care for the hair, caring enough to do the work, and obtaining the required knowledge, seems incredibly difficult for most people. Having healthy hair depends upon your willingness to make the necessary changes. Once you learn the rules they will never change. The better condition your hair is in, the easier it will be to style and the more manageable it will become, all because the hair is healthy. You will kick yourself when you finally realize just how simple and easy it is to grow and keep your hair pretty, healthy, strong and in excellent condition.

You must *make the time* and *do the work* because it is so important. You would be amazed at how many clients want to know why their hair will not grow. They desperately want to find *someway* or *something* to make it grow. The problem is that their hair is falling out faster than it grows, and they are probably getting some very bad haircuts. Nevertheless, it's still growing. You can perm it, rip it out, hot curl it, brush it, chop it off, relax it, color it, or any combination of these things hundreds of times over a life time, and your hair will still grow. It's Growing. So, if you take proper care of your hair, it will grow right down your back.

 A Growing Tip: Do your homework by reading all of the instructions and everything else on the label of every product, before purchasing and again prior to use. The label will tell you everything about the product. Be very careful and follow label instructions exactly.

Realistically, there are some things that can happen by natural causes to change the way the hair will grow and even stop hair from growing. There are things that will change the hair's texture and color. These are things we have no control of, they are just facts of life.

There are illnesses, such as cancer, which requires radiation treatment. This treatment causes hair loss in many patients. There is a condition called Alopecia Areata, which is when the hair comes out in spots, from the size of a dime to the size of a baseball. It could happen at any time and anywhere on the head. It usually leaves the scalp smooth as if there was never any hair there. No one has been able to determine why Alopecia Areata happens or how to get the hair to grow back. In this case, the hair seems to have "a mind of its own" and it comes and goes as it pleases.

Some other reasons the hair falls out are stress, medications, and the aging process. Hair growth is not a continuous process, but it progresses for a period of time, and then it stops. It could change overnight or at any time during your lifetime.

The 100,000 to 150,000 possible hair strands of the scalp are able to grow for years without interruption. Some of us have thin, baby fine hair, while others have thick or very thick hair. Whatever your hair texture or density, live with it, because there is little you can do to grow thicker hair if the follicles are not there.

Shedding periods and baldness occur because of a natural tendency of the follicles (the opening from which the hair extends beyond the scalp) to become very small and possibly even close up as we get older. This could happen anytime after age sixteen. You need not concern yourself with this unless it is a part of your life. Even then, very little can be done about it, short of a hair transplant. Remember, take the time to care for the hair you have because it's growing.

Points to Remember

- ❑ Every chemical service must be done properly and on schedule.
- ❑ Use the right products.
- ❑ Shampoo and condition every four to five days.
- ❑ Always use the best conditioners money can buy.
- ❑ If possible use only one chemical in the hair at a time.
- ❑ If you can afford it, have all of your chemical services done by a professional.

The 24—Month Hair Growth Timetable

This 24-month growth timetable is for people who are chemically relaxing their hair. If you are really serious, and you are willing to do the work, you can grow your hair. This 24-month timetable will help you reach your goal. I have refined the process to insure you will absolutely understand how to make the timetable work for you. The expected growth is approximately a quarter to one half inch per month, and between 10 and 12 inches by the end of the 24 months. This is in addition to the hair you already have. The reason for the estimate of 10 to 12 inches is because some people's hair grows faster than others, and you can expect to have your hair trimmed or cut several times along the way.

This process will only work if you follow the program precisely, make a commitment to do the work and use only the recommended products. I am not saying that other products will not work for this timetable, but based on my experience with the recommend products, I am *positive* they *will* work. Throughout this book I have promised you **real solutions to real problems**, and I do not intend to renege on that promise.

 A Growing Tip: Bleaching, permanent haircolor, curls and relaxers are chemical processes that will cause the biggest changes in the very nature and condition of the hair. Misuse of these products, which happens more often than not, will leave the hair a weird color, dull, spongy, extremely dry and very weak. Even the best conditioners, at this point, will have little, if any, effect. The good thing is that you can start from scratch and replace all of the damaged hair in about 24 to 36 months.

It is best to start with a conditioning program. If you *do not* have permanent haircolor in your hair, use the shampoo and conditioners recommended. If you have been using haircolor for some time and have changed the overall color of your hair and it is unhealthy, stop now. If you have been using haircolor to cover gray hair, you will learn how best to cover gray hair and keep your hair healthy as part of this program.

I will assume you have been using a no-lye relaxer in your hair because most people are using the no-lye relaxer these days. My advice, however, is if you are using no-lye relaxer, STOP using it now and promise never to use it again. The use of No-Lye Relaxer will *not* be a part of this program. If your hair is natural, this same program will work for you and anyone who is not using permanent haircolor and putting it in themselves. This timetable is very simple, so you can relax.

In All of Your Getting, Get Knowledge

The bottom line is keeping the hair healthy, but the secret to your success is education. You must learn the right things to do and when to do them. You must also learn all of the wrong things, which you should not do. Education is the key. Use the best products that will do the best job every time of caring for your hair. Share what you learn with someone else, and God will bless you.

This is How We Do It

Suggested Products

Shampoo Botanoil Treatment from Nexxus:
Formulated for stressed or chemically processed hair. It will strengthen as it improves elasticity, pliability and replenishes essential fatty acids. It is the perfect shampoo to work hand in hand with the conditioner.

Humectress Crème Moisturizing Conditioner:
This conditioner will return more of the needed moisture to the hair with each application. Nothing will soften the hair better.

Always allow the conditioner to remain on, under a plastic cap and under a warm dryer for 15 minutes. Rinse well.

Shampoo and condition every 4 days for the first 4-6 weeks prior to starting this timetable. This is the best way to prepare the hair for starting this program.

During the 24-month timetable, shampoo and condition the hair once a week minimum, do it on the same day if possible, of every week and do not skip a week. You may do more conditioners if you choose, the more the better.

Regardless of the type of relaxer you have been using, your next retouch should be with a **conditioning lye relaxer**. Don't ever return to using the no-lye relaxer. *See a professional for this service.* Continue to use a conditioning lye relaxer and Humectress moisturizing conditioner as your regular conditioner, and stay with it after the 24-month timetable.

The Proper Relaxer for the Retouch

- ❑ This 24-month growth timetable will begin with your relaxer retouch.

- ❑ If this chemical service is to be done at home, remember it takes two people. Never apply the relaxer to your own hair.

- ❑ Use only a conditioning lye relaxer.

- ❑ It is imperative that every time you get a retouch, the chemical is applied to the new growth only.

- ❑ The chemical should never be combed through the hair.

- ❑ The retouch must be done on time every 6 to 8 weeks.

- ❑ If your hair grows fast, it should be done every 6 or 7 weeks, every eight weeks, if your hair grows slowly.

- ❑ If possible have this service done professionally, see The System #1.

A Deep Conditioning Treatment Schedule

KerapHix Crème Reconstructor Conditioner for Stressed Hair:
Rebuilder, reconditioner, strengthens dry, brittle hair. The keratin
protein reinforces the hair's integrity prior to chemical services,
corrects heat damage from thermal appliances, and mends split
ends. The hair should be treated with a deep conditioning protein
treatment every 4th week. This will keep the hair very strong. It
will also give the hair the things it needs that it will not get from the
regular conditioners on a weekly basis.

❑ Have the hair cut or trimmed as needed every six weeks to rid
the hair of split ends. Split ends are the worst kind of breakage. If length is what you are trying to accomplish, it is important to tell your stylist to cut only what is needed to remove
the split ends, about a quarter of an inch in most cases.

❑ When you are growing from short to shoulder length or
longer, the hair will require more work to maintain the style
when the hair is between very short and 8 inches in length.

❑ Apply setting lotion every time before drying the hair. This
will make the hair easier to detangle.

❑ You may hot curl daily with an electric iron if you use
Dudley's Crème Press hairdressing to protect the hair from
the heat. It will also keep the hair nice and soft. Dudley's Total
Control styling spray will help the curls to hold longer. When
you spray on the spritz, comb through the hair and allow the
hair to dry completely; add a smidgen of Crème Press to each
section and curl the hair.

❑ Visit the salon every four weeks to have the hair shampooed
and set, to give the hair a rest from hot curling. This will tie in
with the deep conditioning treatment to strengthen the hair.

❑ You may consider alternating hot curling and roller setting
the hair every other week, if you choose. You will find it to be
much better for your hair. Anytime you can get away from hot
curling and blow-drying it will be better for your hair.

Important Points to Remember

- ❑ Condition the hair every four days for four weeks prior to starting the schedule.

- ❑ The timetable begins with the relaxer retouch.

- ❑ Always use a conditioning lye relaxer, on schedule.

- ❑ Insist that the chemical is applied to the new growth only.

- ❑ Avoid no-lye relaxers altogether.

- ❑ Do a deep conditioning treatment every 4th week including after each retouch.

- ❑ The hair should be conditioned with Humectress weekly.

- ❑ Always use Crème Press hairdressing when hot curling.

- ❑ Alternate hot curling and roller setting every two weeks.

- ❑ Have your hair cut or trim split ends every four weeks or as needed.

- ❑ Repeat the process every eight weeks for 24 months.

- ❑ The 24-month growth timetable should continue throughout your lifetime.

The Proof is in the Pudding

Following this 24-month growth timetable should result in longer, stronger, and healthier hair. It will require discipline and a commitment, but if you truly love your hair and want it to be beautiful, you will do what is required. Follow it explicitly without substitution of any of the **Hair Care Products**. You'll love the results, I promise you. Good luck.

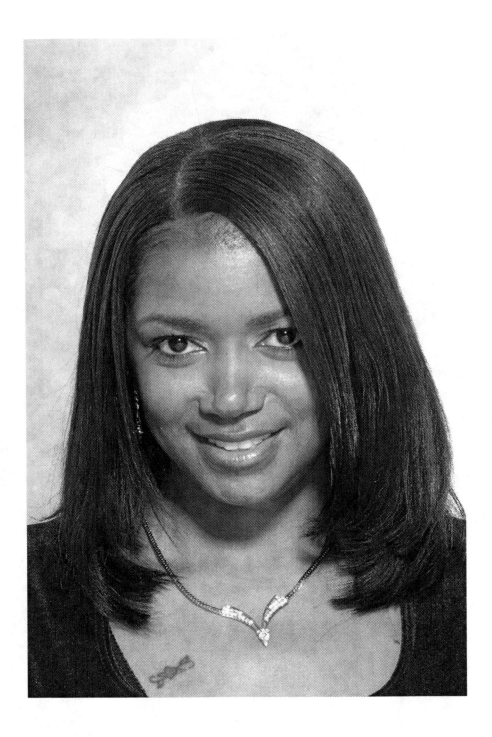

Chapter Three

The Care Package: Real Solutions that Really Work

Hair Styling 101—Just the Basics

One of my most important reasons for writing this book is to help the readers understand why they continue to have a myriad of problems with their hair. The primary reasons are that they break all the rules of proper hair care and chemical application, and they misuse hair products. In addition, some women have a "hands off, do nothing" attitude when it comes to taking care of their hair.

In this chapter, I will share with you the exact way to service your hair from start to finish. You will learn how different hair care products work. Too often we expect the hair care products we use to do more than the job they were designed for. We blame the products for dryness, breakage, inability to hold curl, lack of shine and inability to relax properly. We blame these problems on the product or the hairstylist, but seldom do we blame ourselves, the one really responsible for our hair problems.

The Relaxer and Oil Base

Let's start with the retouch of the relaxer. The purpose for the scalp oil (the base) is not just to place a layer of protection between your scalp and the chemical. The oil base should be a product that is designed for basing the scalp, but it should also be one that will chemically cool the scalp and not block, slow or interfere with the chemical's ability to relax the hair. When applying the base, cover all of the skin that will come in contact with the chemical. This is the purpose for the basing oil.

Remember This If You Don't Remember Anything Else
Cosmetology is a "precise" science. There are exact rules, methods, concepts and ways to do whatever you need to do to your hair. You do not have to guess how to use permanent haircolor, or which relaxer is the right one for your hair. There is no guessing as to how to give your hair the perfect cut, because there are exact ways to cut every hairstyle. You don't have to guess which are the best shampoos, conditioners, setting lotions, setting gels or even who is the best person to style and service your hair. You don't have to guess how long to leave color on, if you should bleach your hair, or how to mix setting lotion.

The Relaxer— Let's Get One Thing "Straight" Right Now

The relaxer has only one job, which is to relax the hair. Notice I did not say straighten the hair—to straighten your hair, relax it. There is a possibility that your hair will be straight after the relaxer. In most cases, this will be a sure thing but only because the conditioning lye relaxer has done its job, which is to rid your hair of its entire natural curl and the hair's natural ability to hold curl. Getting the hair to hold curl after it has been relaxed is easier said than done, unless you know a trick or two. (This will be discussed further in a subsequent chapter).

The chemical destroys all of the natural bonds in your hair. Do not be alarmed by the term "destroy." I use this term to emphasize that once the hair is relaxed, there is no possible way to return that hair to the texture it was before the relaxer, because the bonds have been broken down and chemically exploded into oblivion. It is never necessary to get the hair "bone straight" when relaxing the hair. In fact leaving a little wave in the hair is a much better idea. It will give the hair some natural ability to hold the curl you put in the hair during the styling process.

When the process of chemically relaxing the hair is performed correctly and completed, your hair is permanently relaxed from a curly to a straight position. This is the only job of a relaxer. The fact that the relaxer also conditions as it relaxes your hair is icing on the cake. The addition of conditioners is one of the most wonderful things the makers of relaxers have ever come up with. Product manufactures have done the same with just about every Hair Care Product on the market.

The Bonds of The Hair—Just The Basics

The bonds of the hair are given to us by Mother Nature, and are identical in all forms of hair including human hair, animal and plant hair. We will not get into the vast technicalities of the bonds, however, it is important to know that the greatest portion of bonds in the hair falls under the heading of protein. The major types are the S or sulfur bonds, the H or hydrogen bonds, S-S or disulfide bonds, peptide bonds and chemical bonds.

The bonds determine the structure of the hair, its length, strengths, weaknesses, and its elasticity, which is the hair's ability to stretch and return. The bonds cause the hair to be curly, wavy or straight and help the hair to hold curls naturally when no chemical is present. If the hair is naturally straight, the bonds determine if the hair can be chemically altered to become curly (as with the Curl), and how well it will hold its new curl. The bonds also determine if the hair will be soft, wiry, resistant, or porous. The natural bonds of the hair establish all of these factors and many others.

Special Effects

All hair care products have built within their formulas, properties designed to affect one or more of the bonds of the hair. When these products are used properly, they will have a good effect on those bonds, and the desired results will always occur. To misuse or use the wrong product on your hair could spell disaster because these products will have a very bad effect on the hair.

Every Relaxer Will Do the Same Thing

I had to give some extra thought to what I am about to tell you next, so there will be no confusion. Did you know that every relaxer on the market will do exactly the same thing to your hair, which is relax and straighten it? Notice what I did NOT say. I did not say that every relaxer is the same. They are not the same, and this is where you must be careful in choosing the best and proper relaxer for your hair. It should always be a Conditioning Lye Relaxer. Only the best and the right one for your hair will do.

Your hair will appear to be healthier and very well-conditioned after every chemical service. Permanent haircolor application, the curl, tints and the relaxer retouch all will leave your hair conditioned. However, these are small layers of a conditioning base, none of which will complete the job of fully conditioning your hair. Most hair care products have only one job, the one it is designed for. The ability to condition, to add strength, protein and moisture will be minimal at best, with one exception, the main conditioner product. This is the conditioner that normally follows the shampoo. It is when the conditioners from all of the products you use on your hair are working together that the hair has its best chance to be well-conditioned and become as healthy as possible.

Your Own Conditioning Selection

The job of the main conditioner is to treat the hair, and even that job will vary with different types of conditioners. By the way, when it comes to the main conditioners, any two or three can be used at once. For example, after the chemical service the hair should be treated:

❑ Use a concentrated protein conditioner for twenty minutes under a plastic cap and hair dryer, rinse very well, for a full five minutes. Set a timer.

❑ Apply a crème protein moisturizing conditioner for fifteen minutes, rinse very well.

❑ Spray in a leave-in conditioner, setting lotion, and style as usual.

One of the most important things I hope you will learn from this book is how to choose the right conditioner for the integrity of your hair at the time you purchase the product. It will be necessary to change your conditioner now and then, because your hair will change frequently over time.

Neutralizing Shampoo—The Terminator, My Job Is To Stop You In Your Tracks

The neutralizing shampoo has three jobs. It stops the action of the chemical in its track. This means to stop the chemical from over processing your hair, and nothing else will work. If the action of the chemical is not stopped, it will eat right through your hair. Neutralizing shampoo also normalizes the hair, which means it lowers the pH of the hair. The normal pH of your hair is 7 on the pH scale. When the hair it is chemically relaxed, the pH shoots up to 14, and this pH must be returned to normal or the hair will be very dry. The neutralizing shampoo can do this job also, very well.

The third purpose for the neutralizing shampoo is to thoroughly clean the hair, as you know the hair should never be pre-shampooed the day it is to be chemically relaxed. The cleaning of the hair must take place during the chemical process. If you were to shampoo, get caught in the rain, go swimming or wet the hair in any way and then attempt to dry the hair and get a relaxer the same day, your entire scalp would be on fire in less than five minutes, guaranteed. For this reason you must always tell your stylist if you have wet your hair within 48 hours prior to getting a relaxer.

The thing to keep in mind is that the shampoo, which is part of the formula of this neutralizing product, does not affect the chemical in any way. The shampoo does not wash out the chemical. It will not stop the chemical from working. Only the neutralizer in the shampoo will do that. The neutralizing shampoo will not straighten your hair or cause it to revert back. It will not dry out your hair or cause breakage, and it does not condition. It will only do what any other shampoo will do, which is clean the hair and clear it of dirt, oils, and other debris.

However, its ability to be worked into a thick lather, enables the neutralizer, which is the most important part of the formula, to stay on the hair long enough to terminate the chemical's effect on your hair.

Warning—A "Must Do" Process

The neutralizing shampoo is the most important component in the relaxing process after the hair has been relaxed. If you get this one wrong you could lose all of your hair within one or two weeks, and you may not be able to stop the breakage, so get it right the first time and every time. This chemical relaxer is lye, and it will eat clear through the hair fiber, if the action of the chemical is not stopped. The sad fact is that the action of the chemical is NOT stopped in many cases, at home or in the salon. This is one of the reasons so many of you are having so much breakage.

The Strong Arm of the Conditioner

Hair is 98.9 percent protein, so what kind of conditioner do you want to use most often? You want to use a protein moisturizing conditioner whose job is to give the hair back some of its strength. This is accomplished by infusing the hair with the protein it loses over time and especially after being permanently colored, permed and/or relaxed. The conditioner will also feed the hair and fill it with many of its wonderful natural properties.

 Chemical Tip: Even the best protein conditioners may not stop the hair from falling if you do not allow the neutralizing shampoo to complete its job, of stopping the action of the chemical.

The Water—H2O—The Clear Liquid

Water is like a liquid cargo train and its cargo is everything that needs to take the trip out of the hair. Water is always flowing, on the move, and its only job is to transport and remove product from the hair, except when it's added to a conditioner or setting lotion. The job of water is not to clean the hair. Nor does it neutralize chemicals, enhance haircolor, or condition the hair. Running water on the head for an extended period of time, whether hot, or cool will not make the hair grow. This is a baseless theory that has been circulating but has no merit. The sole responsibility of water is to move product, shampoo, dirt, conditioner, gel, oils and anything else out of the hair.

Water Dilutes or Weakens Product

Water dilutes setting lotion when the two are mixed, and this is very good because setting lotion is concentrated. When water is mixed with neutralizing shampoo, however, this is not good because it weakens the neutralizing shampoo causing it to become less effective. That's why it is so important to towel blot as much water as possible after each rinse. When it comes to the relaxer, water will remove the content of the product itself from the hair, but it will NOT alter the chemical's effect on the hair. Only the neutralizing shampoo will stop the action of the chemical. Don't believe anything to the contrary. (Now pour yourself a glass of cool water, take a couple of sips, and read on.)

Holding Agents

The job of the setting lotion is to soften the cuticle layer so that it will comb easier. It also acts as an artificial bond to help the hair hold its curl in a dry set or when the hair is blown into style with blow dryer and round brush. This set will last two to three days depending on the condition, strength and texture of the hair. Remember that the natural bonds, which caused your hair to hold curl on its own, were destroyed during the relaxing process. If your hair is to ever hold a curl after it has been relaxed, you will need an artificial bonding product. A holding agent such as setting gel, hair spray, spritz, mousse, or setting lotion and a hot curling iron.

There is an abundance of oils, grease and light oil creams on the market simply because everyone in this industry knows that most women of color believe that grease should be used to relieve every kind of hair problem, and dryness is at the top of the list.

Hair Grease and Oils—A-Little-Dab-A-Do-Ya

- ❏ Oil Sheen Spray
- ❏ Oil Sheen Moisturizers, many types
- ❏ Hairdressing
- ❏ Oil Gloss
- ❏ Curling Wax
- ❏ Oils designed just for basing the scalp
- ❏ Hot oil treatment
- ❏ Oil for itchy scalp

The truth of the matter is that hair grease is for the scalp not the hair. It should be used lightly to grease the scalp once or twice a week. It will help keep the scalp soft and pliable.

The hairdressing, on the other hand, should dress the hair with a "sheen," which is a light shine, and it should moisturize at the same time to help keep the hair soft. The other oils can be used on the hair, but should be used very carefully and sparingly. The hair should be shampooed and conditioned at least once a week to remove the oils and the dirt that are attracted to the hair during the course of a normal day.

A Hairdressing Tip

Protection, protection, protection—you must remember this. Crème Press hairdressing by Dudley Products is the one product you should have more of on hand than any other, except conditioner. I can't began to tell you how extremely important it is to use Crème Press hairdressing after, and many times during, every dry set, wet set, and always after blow drying the hair, before hot curling. This product is a must! Crème Press hairdressing will protect the hair from hot irons and will offset any dryness caused by everything else you have used prior to dressing the hair. There is no reason anyone should have dry or very dry and brittle hair when you have Crème Press.

Moisture Retainers

The moisture from each of the products you use, shampoos, conditioners, setting lotions and gels will add some softness, but in varying degrees. However, they do not add enough moisture to protect the hair against the dryness that will occur after the hair is blown dry, wet set and dried under a hood dryer, or hot curled. Your hair will be dry through and through, but this is normal—so relax. A more concentrated moisture retainer will be needed to maintain the hair's softness after it has been serviced and styled. I recommend Crème Press hairdressing, which must be applied lightly and daily to keep moisture and softness in your hair. It will not interfere with the hair's ability to hold curl; actually it will enhance it.

To Sum Up

1. Base the scalp with a protective oil designed for the purpose of basing. I recommend Vitamin AD&E Hair and Scalp Conditioner by Dudley Products.

2. Use a neutralizing shampoo every time, to stop the action of the chemical and return the hair to a normal pH.

3. Use water to rinse well after the chemical, after the neutralizing shampoo, which should be applied and rinsed three times, and after the main conditioner treatment.

4. Spray in some setting lotion to help manage the hair and to give the hair the ability to hold curl. This will also close the cuticle layer, lessening tangles and making the hair easier to comb.

5. Use spritz (Dudley's Total Control), for more holding power, and Crème Press hairdressing for sheen and softness and to protect the hair from hot irons, blow dryers and everyday dryness of the hair.

6. Use a light hair oil to lightly oil the scalp every four to five days. I recommend Vitamin AD&E.

7. Set, style, and enjoy your beautiful hair.

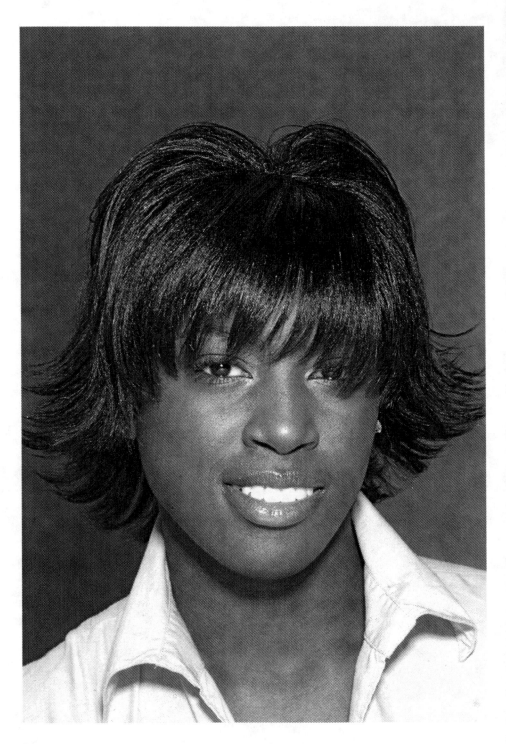

Chapter Four

Stop The Breakage: Putting An End To Dry Brittle Hair

A Magic Potion That Really Works
This Is A Matter Of Extreme Importance

In this chapter I will tell you all about "The Magic Potion," how it works and why it works. I will also tell you about things no one else in the industry will tell you—things you never knew, you never knew. Starting with the "No-Lye Relaxer kit," a silent, man made hair disease, and destroyer. This is one kit you want to leave on the shelf. The chemical in "No-Lye" relaxer causes the hair to become extremely dry. If you have been using this destructive product in your hair or your daughter hair, Stop Now!!! I know, you thought like everyone else that the "No-Lye Relaxer" was better for your hair. That is the real lie and the complete opposite is the undisputable truth. The dryness in hair that this product causes is irreversible, in most cases. The dryness, however, *can* be changed temporarily with the right conditioner, and over time, with the proper care and growth, the damaged hair *can* be replaced.

First-degree burns, to the scalp from the misuse of the Lye relaxer is what has caused woman of color to choose the "No-Lye" relaxer. The error is not with the use of the Lye relaxer, but with the person applying the chemical, and their lack of know-how.

The dryness created by the "No-Lye" relaxer is like a cancer, silently causing the hair to fall out, pieces at a time. Unfortunately, anyone who uses this product, just once, will lose part, if not all, of their hair over a short period of time. The more coarse the hair texture, the more damage the "No-Lye" relaxer will do, and the breakage and hair loss are then accelerated.

THIS IS A VERY DANGEROUS CHEMICAL

A client with very long hair could experience breakage from a ¼ inch to the full length of the hair, at a rate of 50 to 100 pieces per day, which equals 50 to 100 strands per day.

Take a look around. It seems as if most black women are wearing braids or weaves made of synthetic fibers—false hair. These are called hair extensions, meaning they are attached to the hair that is left after the use and misuse of the "No-Lye" relaxer, other chemicals and not properly shampooing and conditioning the hair on a regular basis.

Every product that has the ability to alter the texture and structure of your hair must always be supported with its *complete system*, and only the best. This means you should purchase the *full line* of supporting products. Many people, including cosmetologists, do not read the manufacturer's instructions, and more importantly, will not purchase the required normalizers, shampoos, neutralizing shampoos, conditioners and oils. Many erroneously assume that by substituting or omitting certain products, they can cut costs and save time. Through proper education and training, you *and* your hair care professional can learn the importance of using *a complete product line* in the application of chemical services.

A Fact That Very Few People Know

If you use a "No-Lye" relaxer or home relaxer kit, and take the chemical out of the hair too soon, the hair will not be properly relaxed, and the percentage of curl that is left in the hair will be *locked in the hair*. This product chemically locks the bonds of the hair, preventing anything else from entering the cortex layer, altering its texture. In other words, nothing else, not even another "No-Lye" relaxer will ever straighten this hair. Conditioners, and oil moisturizers will have little or no effect. Your hair will just be extremely dry, and nothing you use will change it except *"The Magic Potion."*

The stronger and more coarse your hair, the dryer, harder and more brittle your hair will become, and dryness is your hair's worst enemy. This kind of dryness pops and breaks the hair in pieces of different lengths. The longer the hair, the longer those pieces will be when the hair begins to silently fall out.

"Even if you use "No Lye" relaxer only once, the dryness, brittle-ness, and breakage are imminent. The more times you use this product, the drier, and more brittle your hair will become and the faster your hair will fall out.

It should take about 2 years to replace the hair that was damaged by the "No- Lye" relaxer. Remember that if the hair is damaged *by anything*, there is no way to return the hair to its *original healthy state*. The most you can do is take the best possible care of your hair, while you grow out of the damaged hair. Whatever you do, don't allow anyone to cut all of your hair off, unless there is absolutely no other solution. FACT! "No-Lye" relaxer causes baldness. Its popularity and the use of it must be stopped in its tracks. Until then, there is a temporary solution—I call "The Magic Potion," or "The Fifteen-Minute Miracle".

Little LaQuida, the Daddy's Girl

This is the true story of how I discovered *The Magic Potion*. Her name was LaQuida, and she was truly a "daddy's girl." Early one Saturday morning, a father came into the salon where I was work-ing , with his daughter, LaQuida. She was a pretty little black girl, about 8 years old, with hair about 14 to 16 inches in length. Her hair was very dry, it had the appearance of burnt charcoal, and it was broken off throughout her head.

LaQuida and her father were concerned that she would lose all of what used to be a *beautiful head of hair*. Someone had put a "No-Lye" relaxer in her hair, probably her first chemical experi-ence. This was in 1989 when I first moved to New Jersey, just after leaving Dudley Cosmetology University in North Carolina.

This was to be the challenge of my career. It was obvious that the father loved his daughter very much. As a father of four Lady

Babies, I certainly understood how he felt, and my heart too was breaking to see what someone had done to LaQuida's hair. When her father asked if there was anything I could do to stop the breakage, I assured him that I would do what I could. This was all very intimidating for me, because I didn't know of anything that would really work. I was not yet aware that a *"Magic Potion"* was awaiting my discovery in the back of the salon.

Marie, the manager of the salon was using the full line of shampoos and conditioners from Nexxus Products at the time.

I looked through the Nexxus product line and found Humectress Moisturizing Conditioner. I used the exact application I have given you in this chapter, and I must admit that I wasn't sure it was going to work. In addition, I used every trick I knew of in my "book of tricks" to service little LaQuida's hair, from start to finish. I used everything I had that contained moisture, the best shampoo, conditioner, crème hairdressing and even a moisture retainer. I prayed, "God please let this work." The old people in my church will tell you, be careful of what you pray for, you might get it. Well, the old folk were right. I told the father to bring LaQuida every week until we could get a handle on the problem.

After 4 or 5 weeks, her hair began to look like new hair. The breakage stopped, the hair was softer, smoother, silkier, and a lot stronger. I was completely "blown away." It was the biggest change I have ever seen take place in anyone's hair in all of my time in this business. After about 2 months, thinking the problem was solved, the father stopped bringing LaQuida to the salon for service. Sure enough, the hair reverted to very dry and brittle, the breakage started all again, and we had to start the whole process over from scratch. So if you are having a similar problem with your hair or your little LaQuida's hair, use The Magic Potion, it is the Real Solution to this very Real Problem of very dry hair.

"The Magic Potion" is Humectress by Nexxus Products

Make a Nexxus connection, and watch it work with Humectress Moisturizing Conditioner from Nexxus Products. This is the only **Hair Care Product** I am positive will work for the dryness caused by the "No-Lye" relaxer and other **Hair Care Products.** Humectress Moisturizing Conditioner is an effective moisturizer for restoring and maintaining the proper moisture balance within the hair shaft. Nothing does it better. Humectress is professionally recommended for home maintenance of dry hair and as a hair moisturizer for all types of hair. Humectress really works, and when used the right way, it will leave the hair soft, silky, and smooth.

This Is How We Do It

It is imperative to follow these directions exactly, with no exceptions:

1. The hair must be very clean. Shampoo the hair at least twice, and be generous with the shampoo.

2. Rinse very well after each shampoo.

3. Towel blot to remove most of the water from the hair.

4. Apply Humectress Moisturizing Conditioner. Use as much as you need, but in quarter size portions, so as not to waste the product.

5. Use a large tooth comb to be sure that the product is equally distributed throughout the hair.

6. Place a plastic cap over the hair, and sit under a warm dryer for twenty minutes.

7. You can purchase a hood dryer for around $50.00. Stay away from the ones with the plastic "shower" caps.

8. Rinse the hair very well. Towel blot, apply a setting lotion, and style as usual.

9. This treatment is a constant, so do it for life! Repeat this exact process every four days for 4 weeks.

10. After 4 weeks, service the hair once every week, if possible, on the same day, and about the same time of day. This will help you to create a regular routine of caring for your hair, and will make sure that the hair is fed on time. It *is not* O.K. to let the hair go a week or two without a good shampoo and Humectress Moisturizing Conditioner.

11. Remember that the hair's ability to return to its dry, brittle state will remain in the hair that has been treated with the "No-Lye" relaxer for as long as that hair remains on your head.

12. Do not stop the treatments and do not change this product for another one because it is the only one that will work. Believe me, I have tried everything else, and nothing else works.

13. You should see and feel a change in the hair after the fourth treatment.

14. The hair should feel very soft, as if the dryness is gone forever, but don't be fooled. The ability of the hair to return to the dryness is still there, but it is under control. Your hair will feel wonderfully silky and look more beautiful than ever, but continue the treatments.

15. The new growth or newly grown hair should be relaxed with a mild or regular strength Conditioning Lye relaxer.

16. From this point on, use only Humectress Moisturizing Conditioner after every shampoo.

17. It should take about two years to replace the hair that was damaged by the "No-Lye relaxer.

Don't Wash Your Hair, Shampoo Your Hair

Always use a professional shampoo that is made especially for use on black hair. This does not necessarily mean a shampoo made by a black **Hair Care Product** company. Selecting the right shampoo is as important as selecting the proper chemicals and conditioners for your hair. A pH-balanced shampoo is a must. When choosing a good shampoo, read the label and look for the term "pH-balanced." It should be understood that neutralizing shampoo, which is normally used after a relaxer application, is *not* a shampoo for everyday cleansing of the hair.

It can be used for that purpose, however, when no other shampoo is available. Remember, it is a *neutralizer*, and the proper application is extremely important. Using a conditioning shampoo or a conditioner and shampoo all-in-one is a very good idea, but should never take the place of the regular conditioning process.

Look for a high quality professional shampoo that contains protein and moisturizers. The shampoo should have a low pH of 4.5 with emollients and cleansers designed to remove oils, product build-up, and dirt from the hair and scalp.

How Often Should You Shampoo Your Hair?

We have all heard that shampooing too frequently is not good for the hair because it strips all of the oils from the hair. Nothing could be farther from the truth. One of the best things you can do for your hair is to shampoo it every four days and even more often, if you choose. Be sure to use a shampoo that is designed for your specific hair type. Whether your hair is oily, dry, color-treated, or normal, there is a shampoo made especially for your hair type. After every shampoo, you must condition the hair. The Nexxus Product Company has the most complete line of shampoos and conditioners on the market.

Conditioners are not designed to be effective after more than five days, therefore conditioning every three or four days will allow the conditioner to build a "conditioning base," causing the hair to become stronger and healthier with each application. The key here is to always use the best product that money can buy.

❑ Clarifying Shampoo

A clarifying shampoo is designed to cleanse the hair thoroughly, while protecting the hair and scalp, even during chemical services. A clarifying shampoo should be used to address special problems such as build-up of residuals from medication, chlorine, hard water, salt-water damage, oil, grease, and other impurities that can be harmful to the hair and scalp. Read the label carefully to choose the right clarifying shampoo for the problem you are having with your hair. Use as directed.

❏ Dandruff Shampoo

This shampoo is different from all other shampoos. It can be used every day, if needed, and use of this product should be continued until the dandruff has cleared up. Dandruff shampoo contains an ingredient that loosens dry and oily dandruff flakes from the scalp, allowing them to be washed away. If the flakes are dry, choose a shampoo to address that problem, and if oily, the same applies. These shampoos are not designed for anything other than treatment of dandruff, and should not be used for problems such as eczema, psoriasis, or other skin and scalp conditions. A dermatologist will be able to treat these conditions, and should be consulted at the first sign of a problem.

 A Gentle Touch Tip: When massaging the scalp, use only the balls of the fingers or the fingertips, but never the fingernails. The fingernails may feel really good, but they also do harm to the scalp. If the scalp is extremely dry and itchy, use the balls of the fingers to apply a light scalp oil designed for that purpose.

Follow the Doctor's Orders

If the dermatologist prescribes a special scalp treatment or shampoo, you and your stylist should follow that treatment regimen explicitly until the problem is resolved. Keep in mind that the *dermatologist* is a *skin specialist*, and is concerned with the scalp, and the *cosmetologist* is a *hair specialist* and is concerned with the hair. Dandruff is often caused by the use of too many chemicals and styling aids or by use of products which are not the right type for your hair and scalp. Everything you use on your hair is a chemical, in one form or another, including water. Even the wrong kind of water will affect your hair.

Let's Talk About Conditioners

What is a conditioner and why should it be used regularly?

- ❑ A conditioner is the key that unlocks the mystery and the secret to beautiful healthy hair.

- ❑ A conditioner is a special chemical agent that is formulated to help restore hair to a natural and healthy state.

There are two major types of conditioners, *non-penetrating* and *penetrating*. The non-penetrating conditioner coats the cuticle layer of the hair with a microfilm coating.

The penetrating conditioner goes deep into the cortex layer of the hair shaft to restore vital proteins. Both types can be used at the same time, and in many cases, they should be.

This Is How We Do It

The best conditioners contain concentrated levels of protein and moisture.

1. After every shampoo, rinse very well, and apply a good conditioner.

2. Cover the hair with a plastic cap, and sit under a dryer for 15 minutes or at room temperature for 25 minutes.

3. Conditioners containing concentrated levels of protein are *not* suitable for hair that is very dry or hair that has been treated with a "No-Lye" relaxer.

4. If one is used in your hair, rinse very well for a full five minutes especially around the face and hairline, where the hair is normally very dry from water and soap scum of daily washing of the face.

5. Apply a heavy high quality *cream moisturizing conditioner*. Always pay close attention to the hairline.

6. Set a timer, and let the conditioner sit for a full twenty minutes.

7. Rinse again very well, apply some setting lotion and style as usual.

The surface of the hair shaft is very similar in appearance to the scales on a fish, overlapping, tight, shiny and slippery when the hair is healthy and wet. The hair fiber has a translucent protein outer layer consisting of seven to twelve cuticle cell structures, and when they are very badly damaged, the hair can never be returned to its original healthy state. However, high quality conditioners, which should always be used, will help keep the hair in its most healthy condition.

High quality conditioners, when used regularly, will reduce cuticle roughness and help the hair be stronger, comb easier, shine, and feel softer. The conditioner will leave a microfilm coating on the hair, and counteract static electricity so that the hair will be more manageable.

There are many different types of conditioners on the market, and most are designed for a specific purpose. Not all are quality conditioners, and those that are not should be avoided. The secret to success in treating your hair is in choosing just the right conditioner for the specific hair problem you are experiencing. Always use the best that money can buy. You may say this is easier said than done, but it is much easier than you think. Later in this chapter, we will discuss some of the many different conditioners. We will find out what they do, how they work, and how best to choose them and use them. The list is endless.

The Problem of Dryness Caused by the Use of No-Lye Relaxers

This is by far the most crucial piece of information I will offer in this book, and it is the one I am more passionate about than any other. Finding the solution has been a personal challenge for me for more than twenty years, and it is one of the most difficult hair care problems facing women of color today. It is one for which there seemed to be no solutions, until now. The questions you may ask are, "why is my hair so dry?" "Why is my hair coming out by the handful?" "What can I do to stop my hair from breaking?"

In my research for this book, it came to light that hair loss is an issue of utmost concern for women of color everywhere, and it can be very scary. The average black woman will find that almost every female she knows, young and old, is dealing with the devastating problem of dry hair and breakage. Unfortunately, there are unscrupulous people out there who do not care about your hair. They are the makers of cheap products and they use the lowest level of raw materials available to make them. They are not concerned about the fact that their products don't work because they know the consumer will buy them.

In the marketplace high quality and very high quality conditioners can be found. There are also low quality and very low quality products. Many of you have been purchasing and using the lower quality products. These are usually very inexpensive, they don't work, and they were never designed to work.

A Common Sense Tip:

Whatever you do, don't let anyone talk you into cutting off all of your hair simply because your hair is damaged, unless there is no other course of action. Also know this, the shorter hair will never out grow the longer. All of the hair will grow at about the same rate, a ¼ to a ½ inch per month. You should get the hair shaped or trimmed occasionally, and after a few months the hair should be about the same length all over.

Concentrated Protein Conditioners

Conditioners containing concentrated levels of protein should always be rinsed very well, for about 5 full minutes, especially around the hairline, and face. (Set a timer) The hair around the hairline, and face is usually very dry from the daily use of facial soaps, which are not designed for use on hair. This leaves the hair around the face dry. In most cases, the texture is weaker than the hair in the crown and the back of the head, and since it is already fragile, the breakage will begin in this area.

Designed to build strength, concentrated protein conditioners harden the cuticle layer. If you rinse this conditioner well but do not add an additional moisturizing conditioner, drying and styling the hair will create a straw-like texture, and the hair will simply break and fall out.

Keep in mind, when choosing conditioners, they should be right for your particular hair condition and type. For example, if you are conditioning very porous hair (color treated, hair that has a curl or relaxer in it, or hair that is very damaged) a very high quality protein conditioner should always be used to help rebuild and strengthen the hair. This, of course, is not the conditioner that contains concentrated levels of protein, but normal levels of protein. Heavy crème moisturizing conditioners should be avoided for this type of hair because they will only cause hair in this condition to become even softer and heavier. They will leave the hair limp, and getting the final set to hold curls will be very difficult at best. Instead of a moisture treatment, choose a quality protein pack.

Types of Concentrated Conditioners

Protein treatments, reconstructors, revitalizing protein packs, rejuvenators, and deep penetrating treatments, are all concentrated protein conditioners designed to strengthen the hair. It is very important to use these conditioners with caution, in fact, they should be done in the salon, by a professional. If they are not rinsed very well, they could do more harm than good. Follow up with a heavy moisturizing conditioner, and only use this kind of conditioning treatment when necessary.

A Treatment Scenario

You have come to the salon for a treatment because you are experiencing breakage from extreme dryness. Most stylists will reach for a concentrated protein conditioner, which is designed to stop breakage. It will harden, strengthen, and rebuild the cuticle layer of the hair. Think about what is happening if your hair is already dry, brittle, and it's breaking. A concentrated protein conditioner will add to the problem and cause even more damage, and breakage.

This means that if these conditioners are applied to hair that is already dry and brittle, the dryness doubles or even triples, which will also double the amount of breakage. Although it is best to have these types of treatments performed in the salon, if you must do this at home, there are a few things to keep in mind. Concentrated conditioners will stop most hair breakage, but they should never be used on hair that is very dry and brittle to stop breakage caused by that dryness. There is such widespread use of the "No-Lye" relaxer, only a good heavy moisturizing conditioner will work in this case—*"The Magic Potion."*

In every other case where dryness is not a problem, a concentrated protein treatment can be applied every time you see more shedding or breaking than normal and after every chemical service, which is about every 6 to 8 weeks.

❑ Normal shedding is about 50 to 100 small pieces to full strands of hair a day.

❑ The most important thing to remember is that concentrated protein conditioners should be rinsed for five full minutes, or until the hair feels smooth, soft and silky to the touch.

❑ Set a timer, then while rinsing, pay close attention to the hair around the face. It is normally more dry, and fragile than all of the other hair. Add an extra portion of moisturizing conditioner in this area.

Moisturizers and Moisturizing Conditioners

The majority of **Hair Care Products** made for women of color contain moisturizers. Moisturizers are found in relaxers, curls, setting lotion, oils, creams, hairdressing, haircolor of all types, and many other products. The one thing that black hair lacks more of than anything else is moisture, which simply means softness, not wetness, and it is always what you are trying to accomplish while servicing your hair. The same is true even if you are wearing a dry set, and if the hair is hot curled.

A Hair Rebuilder

The name says it all. Hair Rebuilders are conditioners formulated utilizing moisturizing conditioners, panthenol, protein and other effective moisturizers for restoring and maintaining the proper moisture and protein balance within the hair shaft. (Dry Brittle Hair Excluded)

This is the conditioner I recommend for use on a regular basis. The protein/moisture balance in this product is always just right for everyday use. Since the hair is made up of about 98% protein, the Hair Rebuilder is the perfect conditioning treatment. It restores protein as it inhibits moisture loss. Hair Rebuilders are perfect for the home maintenance of normal dry hair. If you have a relaxer in your hair, which should always be a conditioning lye relaxer, or if you have a relaxer and permanent haircolor in your hair, I recommend a Hair Rebuilder.

Permanent haircolor and Hair Rebuilders work well together. This conditioner was designed to rebuild badly damaged hair. There is a treatment with every application of this product. The key is to use it often, don't change it for another conditioner ever and don't stop using the product. There are several of them on the market.

This is How We Do It

- ❑ The hair should be shampooed twice, then rinsed very well.
- ❑ Towel blot the hair after each rinse to remove excess water.
- ❑ The conditioner should be applied in quarter-size portions.
- ❑ Use as much as you need, but only in quarter-size portions.
- ❑ Use a large tooth comb, to comb the conditioner through to ensure all the hair is covered.
- ❑ Place a plastic cap over the head, and set a timer for ten to fifteen minutes.
- ❑ The product will actually work in five minutes, if time is a problem.
- ❑ Rinse very well, every time.

❑ Spray in setting lotion to make the comb-out easier.

❑ Dry the hair, apply some hairdressing and styling spray.

❑ Set and style as usual.

Leave-In Conditioner

A leave-in conditioner speaks for itself and can be used as often as you choose. However, the leave-in conditioner does not take the place of the regular conditioner. The process should be: shampoo, rinse, apply regular conditioner, rinse, apply leave-in conditioner, apply setting lotion, and style as usual. The leave-in conditioner can be mixed with setting lotions or sprayed in before every comb out and set.

Crème Rinse

Many times after a shampoo and conditioner, the hair tangles very badly, like putting two pieces of Velcro together. Cream rinse softens the hair, making it easier to comb. The cream rinse is not good for much else. It works instantly, and it coats the hair, which is why it should be rinsed very well. Setting lotion will do exactly the same thing. The cream rinse should be used after the rinse of the regular conditioner.

All In the Family

Purchase the same line of product for all your shampoos, conditioners, setting lotions, oils, sprays, gels and so on, if possible—it's a family affair. They are formulated to work together, which is better for your hair. If a particular line of products does not carry a product you may need to address a specific problem, then purchase what you need from another line. However, make sure it is a high quality product.

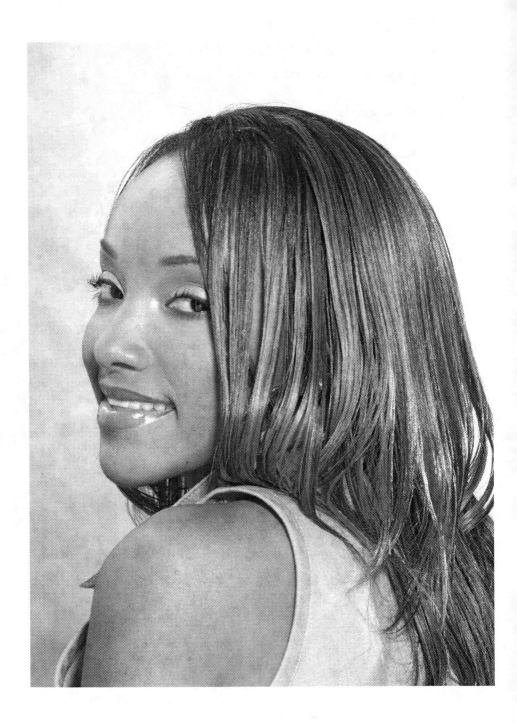

Chapter Five

It's A Natural Thing: Natural Hair, Extensions, Weaves, and Wigs

Your hair is most healthy when it is in a natural state. Whenever chemicals of any kind are applied, they change the hair completely. Those changes are irreversible and that hair is no longer natural in texture. The perfect opportunity for the hair to remain healthy is when it is free of chemicals. The hair is strongest when it is natural, but you must do what is required to keep it that way. You have many choices to make, and those choices will determine the condition of your hair now and throughout your lifetime. You must select the best shampoos, conditioners, and other maintenance products that will keep your natural hair beautiful and healthy.

Hair is Hair

Perhaps you have decided to discontinue the use of chemicals. That is good. However, it doesn't change the importance of using the best shampoos and conditioners to protect, strengthen, and keep your natural hair healthy. If you do a poor job caring for your natural hair, then discontinuing the use of chemicals will be of no benefit. Natural hair is just hair, and the only thing that will change is that you will be wearing your hair natural and free of chemicals. You must still condition your hair every week like clockwork.

I am concerned about the health of your hair and that you don't get so carried away with the term "natural" that you leave yourself open to everything that is labeled "natural." The emphasis should be on the quality of the product rather than whether it is considered a "natural" Hair Care Product or not. There are some very good natural Hair Care Products in the marketplace,.

Hair Horrors and Wacky Remedies from Cyber Space
Double Click on Far-Fetched

Cyber Space (the Internet) has become a place where women visit in search of answers to a variety of hair-related questions. Some black hair care websites receive thousands of "hits" everyday. There are discussion groups and chat rooms where people are talking about black hair all of the time. You can get advice on how to have it your way, how to relax it, be natural, how to make your own conditioners, oils and such. Lively open dialogue is great, but the problem is that much of what is being shared is misinformation that is misleading and confusing.

People are passing along "wacky" remedies and sharing homemade concoctions thinking that they are helping each other out. Most are just ordinary folk, although some of them are hair care professionals, most are not. They are mothers, college coeds, career women and others, who chat "in disguise" using pseudonyms such as "Dominican Girl," "Onelove," "KJ," "Pookipooh," "Weaverbeliever," and my favorite, "Anonymous." Then there are those that I like to call the "undiscovered kitchen chemists." They are the ones that share their weird hair care concoctions on-line. You've got to love these lovely ladies of color. They try hard, but don't be fooled into using that stuff on your hair. You could end up as bald as I am!

Everyone seems to be talking about hair. Sure, visiting these chat rooms and even participating in the discussion groups can be interesting and even fun. However, don't take everything that is said there to be fact. There are so many horrors stories and wacky remedies floating around out there, but you must be wise and always seek advice from hair care professionals.

If It Says "All-Natural"—Is That Good?

I am what you may call a "night person," which means that when most people are asleep, I am wide-awake. I get to watch a lot of infomercials on TV, because they usually come on in the wee hours of the morning. I always pay close attention to anything related to hair. Most amazing are the products that appear on the scene making outlandish claims and promises. These "new discoveries"

The Chit-Chat

"I've found that if you stand in the shower and allow hot water to just run on your head for 20 to 30 minutes, it will speed up the growth of your hair. If that doesn't work, oil the ends of your hair."

"I feel that conditioning the hair is a total waste of time." (Try this one and I promise we will look like twins).

"For daily moisture I spray my hair every day with warm water."

"I heard that there is a pill consisting of 2,000,000 mgs that promises to grow six inches of hair in six weeks. Does anyone know where I can buy it?" (*Now that's really funny*)!

are always packaged attractively and they are usually endorsed by some well-known celebrity.

Their vigorous advertising campaigns initially result in substantial sales. However, after a short period of time, these products disappear. The truth is that when the infomercial disappear, it is because these products have caused severe damage to consumers' hair, forcing their removal from the market. Remember, use extreme caution when considering the use of new products that make outrageous claims.

An All-Natural Wacky Remedy—Can You Trust It?

It is my intent here to show what could possibly go wrong if your only criteria for selecting a Hair Care Product is based upon the descriptive wording on its packaging, such as "all natural," or "no-lye," or "completely safe." Should you be able to trust what they say? The answer is yes, but can you? Not always.

One day a few years back one of my clients called about a real problem her sister was having. The sister's hair was coming out by the handful. My client wanted me to see if anything could be done to stop this. When the sister came to the salon, what I saw was frightening. All of her hair, from an inch above her ears and down, was completely gone, except her very short new growth. In some places, you could even see patches of her scalp.

I lifted pieces of the hair she had left on top, which was about eight to ten inches in length. It came out with very little tension, and I realized it wouldn't be long before she would be completely bald. Reluctantly, she confessed that she had ordered XYZ and used it on her hair. She tried to justify her actions by saying, "They said it was all natural and chemical free. They promised I would never need to use chemicals again. They promised it was perfectly safe. The man even ate some of it!"

I knew there were no answers, no real solutions to this one, but I was willing to try. A chemical relaxer was out of the question. My very best conditioners, which normally worked for every other problem of breakage, did not work this time. During the shampoo, conditioning, and detangling processes, the hair continued to come out by the handful. I gently set the hair on rollers and added a small amount of moisture, so that the hair would dry soft. In the final comb-out, the hair was still falling, and when I styled it, her hairstyle looked like a helmet. She had no hair all the way around her head from the top of the ears down. What she really needed was a serious haircut, but she became angry with me every time I made that suggestion. I wanted to tell her, "Please don't tell any-body that I did your hair." (This was the ugliest hairstyle I have ever done).

After two to three weeks of my trying to stop the breakage, and her trying to style her hair at home, this pretty lady decided to switch to the next stylist in the salon. After she switched, she immediately agreed to have her hair cut into a short, but lovely, hairstyle. I had never been so happy to see a client leave my chair in my life.

One Size Fits All

One of the problems with such products as XYZ is the "one size fits all concept," which is absolutely impossible. Everyone's hair is different in condition, health, and strength. No two people have the same texture of hair, and most have many different textures on the same head. Their hair has been treated with various shampoos, coloring systems and dissimilar relaxer formulas, all of which must be taken into account. Whatever the mixture of possibilities, it all must be added to the XYZ formula, and that is where the statement that *it is safe* begins to unravel.

Instead of relaxing your hair as it promises, the product eats away at the hair fiber. It eats tiny holes into every strand, very much like bleach does if you try to go to blonde, which is at Level 10, from the color black or darkest brown, which are at Level 1 and Level 2. Whatever else it does, it has to alter the chemistry of your hair completely and permanently. It has to have an effect on the bonds and other properties of your hair in order to work.

Stunt the Hairdresser

Such damage creates the only situation I have ever encountered where I believe the only real solution is to cut all of the hair off or at least very short. All of the properties, everything that makes it hair, have deteriorated to nothing. When the hair shaft is reduced to such a fragile, weak and mushy state, it has been damaged to the point of no return. The only thing left to do is to start from scratch and grow a new head of hair.

All of the hair will eventually come out. The same thing will likely happen with the use of no-lye relaxer, bleach, and one of the curl systems in the marketplace. The hair has been reduced to a dry, hard, straw-like substance, just the opposite of healthy, as promised. The breakage can occur over a long or short period of time.

A Final 911 Note

To attempt to return to using a chemical relaxer after a product like XYZ, or even to apply relaxer to natural hair that has been treated with XYZ, will almost instantly take out all of the hair. The same thing will happen if you use bleach and apply a relaxer, or if you are wearing a curl and you permanently change your haircolor and apply a chemical relaxer. The latter is called "triple processing," which will *guarantee* hair loss. (Double click on "meltdown.")

The Big Secret

Remember this one and it will change everything for you and your hair, but please *don't keep this secret to yourself*. In fact, tell everyone you meet. Did you know that most of the natural ingredients found in "natural" Hair Care Products are also found in "regular quality" Hair Care Products? Would you be surprised to learn that the makers of the very best conditioners, shampoos, light crème oil moisturizers with protective properties, and even haircolor, have been making their full line of products this way for many years?

Quality Hair Care Products Are Also Designed For Natural Hair

- ❑ They are not designed to do harm to natural hair.
- ❑ They are wonderfully designed to take the very best care of your hair.
- ❑ The top conditioners and shampoos will never dry out the hair.
- ❑ They are full of moisturizers, protein and other natural oils.
- ❑ The best products will never cause damage, breakage, clog the pores, or restrict hair growth in any way.
- ❑ Instead they build strength and protect the hair.
- ❑ The best ones are considered to be natural food for the hair.
- ❑ They contain many of the natural properties ordinarily found in human hair, that were put there by Mother Nature, which is one of the reasons they work so well.
- ❑ When you buy and use cheap products, you get what you pay for, and your hair will pay even more in the end.

Only the Right One is the Exact One

When purchasing products for your hair, whether your hair is natural or relaxed, you must know exactly what each one does, and that product must do what it promises. You should know exactly how to use each product for the best results. Each of the products you select must be the exact one for the needs of your hair. Each one must work every time with no compromises and no exceptions. I know that it is easier said than done, but this book was written to help you make informed decisions about hair care.

If you do things the right way, whether it is coloring the hair, relaxing, or shampooing and conditioning, your hair will be stronger, healthier and a lot better looking. Remember, hair is hair. The fact that your hair is free of chemicals doesn't change a thing. The hair still has to be shampooed and conditioned on a regular basis with top of the line Hair Care Products or you will have problems with your hair.

Time For an Oil Change

I would like to dispel the misconceptions about the use of oils and grease. Some Hair Care Professionals will disagree, but the truth speaks for itself. Over many years the makers of Hair Care Products have sold the black woman enough heavy oils, grease and petroleum to fry enough chicken to feed all of the State of Texas.

This whole thing with grease and black hair has been around forever. Grease was used in the early days with hot combs and curling irons. Lard and animal fat was used to make the first lye relaxers, and even soaps for doing the laundry and bathing.

I have been teaching about hair for many years, and the way I like to teach is by being as exact and as simple and to-the-point as possible, so as to not mislead or confuse anyone. There are many of you who seem to think that the way to end the dryness in your hair is to *oil it*. The fact is you may have been using the wrong kinds of oils and using them the wrong way.

I think it's time for an "oil change." Some people will use anything, as long as it says "oil," on their hair—homemade concoctions, "a little of this and a little of that." Why would anyone use olive oil, rosemary, eggs, mayonnaise, vinegar, lemon juice or apple cider, to condition the hair and scalp? (Double click on oil is for dummies.)

Heavy oil moisturizers were meant for use on the curl, and are not suitable for dry hairstyles. Many women are using heavy hair grease, petroleum jelly, and the all time favorite, hot oil treatments, to relieve dryness. I have never seen any reason for a hot oil treatment. I'm sure that is surprising to many people. The reason is that it takes forever to get such heavy oil out of the hair. That being the case, why use it in the first place?

 An Oil Tip: The percentage of oil in quality Hair Care Product formulas is added in minimal portions. These are refined very light oils, not heavy, as with olive oil and hot oil treatments. Other conditioners, protein, moisturizers, softeners, lanolin, crèmes and fragrances, are also added to the formulas, which further reduces the overall portions of oil. These ingredients and others are included in the formulas of chemical relaxers, curl re-arrangers, shampoos, conditioners, haircolor, and crème hairdressing.

My Explanation

The reason I say that oil and grease are not for the hair is because, if I were to say otherwise many of you would misuse or over use oil. You must change your way of thinking. If you purchase the wrong types of oils and apply them the wrong way, this will place your hair right back in a dry and greasy condition.

When You Add It All Up

❑ It is the designed combination of all of these wonderful ingredients that when applied will reduce dryness in your hair plus give you the best possible chance of keeping your hair healthy.

- ❑ Maintenance products can be applied daily with no build-up on the hair.
- ❑ Cream hairdressing moisturizes, softens and adds sheen in one step.
- ❑ Conditioning shampoos cleanse the hair and moisturize in one step.
- ❑ When these oils are bottled or put in jars, clear with no additives, they should be so light that if you were to apply them to the back of your hand, they would seep into your skin.
- ❑ Hair color, relaxers and curl re-arrangers condition during application.
- ❑ All of the oils used in good products are extracted from sources conducive to enhancing the overall health, strength and protection of your hair.
- ❑ If these sound like the perfect products for use on natural hair, they are. Nothing is better.

Your Oil Light Is On, Check Your Oil

The opposite of dry is wet, which means that the answer to dryness is not oil, but moisture. Oil expands with heat. Try this. Drop a tiny drop of oil on a piece of colored cloth. Leave it for about twenty minutes then check it. You will find that it has expanded to about the size of a quarter. Oil does the same thing when applied to your hair. In a very short period of time the hair will suck up the oil like a sponge. If the oil is heavy, it fills the hair leaving it limp, gooey and greasy-looking, with an unclean appearance.

Removing the oil and keeping the hair and scalp clean could be very difficult. Imagine trying to shampoo dreads, braids and locs that have been soiled with heavy oils. Imagine how unclean both the hair and scalp can become.

Why Oil Should Be Used Sparingly

When I first started to work with The Dudley Products Company, I had a problem understanding how to use the many oils, crèmes, oil sprays and liquids the company makes. One day I met Pam, a hairstylist who had been with the company about two years before me.

I was the only male stylist with the company, and getting the girls to talk with me about hair wasn't easy at first. So one day I said to Pam, "I am having a very difficult time with the oils. My finished looks are heavy and greasy-looking."

Pam told me to use very little of the oils, and to use them in very small dime-size portions. Just a very light film coating, a smidgen, would do the job. She explained that each of the oils is different and each is used for a different reason. Using the oils in small portions will allow you to use as much as you need without overdoing it. So don't overdo it. Learn the job of each oil, and use them only for those purposes.

When she told me this, suddenly there was magic, and I began to turn out some of the most beautiful hair ever, with a natural looking shine and brilliance, never too heavy, even with the Curling Wax, which is the heaviest of all the oils. Think of the way you apply the oils as tiny, like the strands of hair. Just a little will do the job.

The Curling Wax was the most difficult to use because it is so heavy. If you use Curling Wax the right way, it is perfect for use when starting locs. Dudley's Curling Wax is not the same as Bee's Wax, so don't be concerned about the build up. This oil can easily be broken down and shampooed out of the hair with any good clarifying shampoo.

The Crème Press hairdressing turned out to be the most wonderful light creamy oil I have ever used on black hair. It is the only thing you will ever need to use on dry hair, and it is especially perfect for natural hair textures, dreadlocks, braids, cornrows and other natural hairstyles.

Why Crème Press for Natural Hairstyles?

❑ It is so good for natural hair because it acts as a softening agent, lubricating, which means to moisturize and relieve dryness in medium to coarse hair, especially natural hair, no matter how dry the hair is.

❑ Crème Press can be used every day.

❑ It never leaves a heavy finish, and many of its ingredients are also natural.

❑ The content washes out easily, even after a week of applying daily.

Then there is the Vitamin AD&E, a very light oil which can be used for basing the scalp before applying a chemical relaxer. It will not interfere with the chemical's ability to perform. The Vitamin AD&E is also the light oil you should use to lubricate the scalp, but use it lightly. It can be used on chapped lips, on the body when your skin is dry, and it is great for your hands and feet. Its molecules are so small, when used lightly, they seep into the skin. You should use this product every four days on your scalp.

The Scalp Special is a medicated, minty, light oil that is perfect for itchy scalp when used lightly.

The Oil Sheen Spray is a light oil with the same vitamins found in AD&E. It is a perfect sheen for the finished look and where the hair is tightly curled, kinky or natural.

Just Weave It

"When I was seventeen, it was a very good year," and weave could only be obtained if you were to travel from my hometown of Goldsboro, North Carolina to New York City, which we referred to as "going up the road," in those days. Very few women wore weaves then, and the cost was $150 to $200 for a full head of human hair. When a black woman wore a weave or a wig at that time, it was a well-kept secret. For many years women of color were ashamed to let it be known they were wearing weaves and wigs. Today, it has become commonplace. So many women are wearing false hair, grandmothers, mothers, teens, and even little girls, and that is very sad..

This form of styling the hair has gone through somewhat of a metamorphosis over the years. In many salons today weaving or some other form of hair attachment service, accounts for more than 60% of the salon's business. This is because so many women have lost so much of their own hair from the misuse of chemicals and other things, which has resulted in severe damage.

With so many methods of attaching the hair, it is possible today to wear a different hairstyle every day of the week.

A Real Deal or What?

I have a friend in Chicago who dedicates all of her time to weaving hair. She uses a concept called "strand-by-strand," which is a method of weaving that produces results that are virtually unde-tectable and very natural-looking. A full head of weave using this method and real hair can cost from $800.00 to $2,000.00, and takes many hours to complete.

A Life Saver for Bad Hair Days

If you are considering some type of hair alternative such as a weave, braids, or hair extensions, also consider a quality human hair wig. There are many very good wigs on the market today, and some of them are made so well that no one would ever know you were wearing a wig. Make sure the wig or hairpiece you choose is human hair, and be sure it looks as much like your real hair as pos-sible. If you buy two or three wigs just alike, and one or two differ-ent ones, you will never have another "bad hair day." Choose a style similar to the way you normally wear your hair, then no one will ever know the difference.

For a Limited Time Only

It will only take one to three years to grow a full head of healthy hair using the solutions and methods for hair recommended in this book. No matter what the present condition of your hair is, and regardless of the length of your hair, and the extent of the breakage, with a little patience, a sincere desire, and a willingness to do what is required, you can have a beautiful healthy head of hair. It really is possible. This means that you should consider the weave or wig on a temporary basis only.

Human Hair vs. Synthetic Hair vs. Real Hair

Human hair, is no substitute for your real hair, and you must put all of your focus, energy, and desire into the belief that your own hair can be beautiful. You must clear your mind of every negative thought that such a thing is impossible, because it is possible, and you can do it. I see some of the most beautiful black women God has ever created, and it blows my mind to see that they have lost so much hair that they have to wear weaves. I have to admit, I really don't understand.

It is not always easy, but if you and a very good stylist work together, there is absolutely no reason why you can't grow and have your very own beautiful hair. You will actually find that not only will your real hair be lovelier than ever, it will be easier to manage and care for than a weave, braids or other alternative. Plus, it will cost you a whole lot less money.

Wash and Wear Hair

If you have made up your mind to get a weave hairstyle, it should start with the proper hair. Remember, not all hairstylists are proficient in weaving techniques and methods, so select the stylist to perform this service very carefully. Most of the time, the stylist will choose synthetic hair because it can be purchased for very little money. By doing so, the stylist can charge the client a price that is reasonable, and still make a decent profit. If you are not willing to spend three or four hundred dollars to have your hair weaved, you are probably not working with a pro, and that person is probably not using real hair.

Human hair works the same as your own hair, with a few exceptions. In fact, it works better because it can and should be shampooed and conditioned as often as your real hair. The texture most often is of very high quality, and you know by now how I feel about quality. There are two types of human hair on the market that are most popular, Chinese and Indian hair, which are better than most and look beautiful and healthy. It is important that the hair is double-density, 100% human hair. I recommend that you do not leave the job of buying the hair solely to your stylist. Make the purchase yourself through her, but be prepared to spend a little more money. The Internet will have many suggestions.

Double Click on Possibilities

Human hair comes in many colors, lengths and textures from long to short, curly, wavy and straight. It can be cut to any shape and style, as long as you keep in mind that it is a weave, and it won't grow back. Human hair can be shampooed, conditioned, colored, permed, relaxed, blow-dried, and styled as easy as your own hair. It will not tangle easily unless it is in poor condition. When properly cared for, it will remain soft, beautiful, and manageable.

Color Me the Colors of the Rainbow

Today, synthetic fiber is widely used. However, synthetic fiber will melt with too much heat, and it does not look or feel like real hair, at least when the attachments are first put in. One of the most beautiful things I see from time to time is the use of permanent haircolor and bleach—gorgeous reds, golden browns and blondes. Every color of the rainbow is available.

The use of these chemicals changes the texture of synthetic hair fibers. They swell the synthetic fibers and give the hair a more real and natural appearance. There are numerous choices of curl configurations that come from the manufacturers already permanently locked into the fibers, and will hold the curl as well after coloring. You might consider using haircolor and bleaching.

There are some drawbacks to wearing a weave, braids and other attachments. Here are a few to consider. In order to maintain and care for your new weaved hairstyles, every two months or so you will still have to return to the salon for service. Your real hair will still be growing at the scalp, and it will need to be relaxed as usual.

The weave will have to be removed and put in again. The good news is that you won't have to purchase new hair every time.

The cost of each return visit could be between $50 and $100 less than when the hair was first weaved. Of course this price will vary according to your stylist. If the stylist didn't do a good job, you could have a number of other problems such as matting, the hair coming loose and falling out, or the texture could be all wrong and removing the hair could cost you a bit of your own hair.

Natural Hairstyling Possibilities

Braids, Cornrows large and small, Dreadlocks, net weaving for bald spots, Micro Braids, Kasamas Braids, Pyramid Braids, Twistlocks, Interlock Braids and Janju Braids are some of the many styles. Use human hair, synthetic hair, or your own hair, and any one of these will look great. Keep in mind that everyone's real natural hair texture is not suitable for these natural hairstyles because some hair may be too thin, too fine or too soft.

Leave it to the Professionals

The best way to get started is to find a qualified professional, and spend the money needed to get it right. You will need all of the help you can get, and at the top of your list of needs will be the need for patience. It will take some time, but it will be worth every minute to have your beautiful natural hairstyle. So be patient.

Synthetic Hair

I know it won't do a lot of good to say to you, "don't go there," because sometimes how much money you can spend will dictate. However, the thing about cheap, synthetic hair is that it never looks like real hair. It tangles very badly, wads up, and can be almost impossible to manage. It is hot, hard to keep clean, and looks like false hair. Some textures are better than others, so be selective.

The saddest thing I see just about everywhere I travel is the many black women of all ages who are wearing synthetic braids. You can even buy synthetic braided wigs. Now that's going far enough.

Grooming Natural Hair

Before any grooming enters the picture there is a complication. Depending on the hair's natural style, shampooing and conditioning the hair can be very difficult. The problem is that when you are wearing braids, cornrows and other natural styles, including synthetic hair, there is the possibility of locs becoming undone, or braids slipping loose and coming out. Perhaps you think "if my braids are not real hair it doesn't make sense to shampoo or condition them."

This is absolutely wrong. Since your real hair is also a part of the equation, it becomes the very reason a good shampoo and a very good conditioner are vital to maintain its health. The process is a constant, which means you must shampoo and condition regularly, no exceptions. In terms of the natural hair, locs or otherwise, being long, thick and more difficult to clean doesn't change a thing. Perhaps you are thinking that rinsing shampoos and cream conditioner will be troublesome to manage, or that creamy conditioners will cause a buildup on the hair and scalp. You are both right *and* wrong, but it doesn't change a thing. You still have to shampoo and condition regularly with very good products, no exceptions.

The reason some shampoos and conditioners leave a buildup is because they coat the hair. They are designed to make you think they have done wonders for your hair and that they have corrected many of the problems with weak, lifeless and dry hair. These are mostly cheap products so stay away from them. The solution is quality hair care products. They can be removed as easily as they are applied, plus they will keep the hair as healthy, strong, and as beautiful as possible. To not shampoo and condition regularly will result in creating problems with your hair such as dryness, hair breakage, and damage to the cuticle and cortex layer. The thing to remember is that once the hair is damaged it cannot be undone.

Keeping Natural Hairstyles Clean, Strong, and Moisturized

So let's solve all of the problems with shampooing and conditioning natural hair. Purchase a hair net, one that has small wholes in it like a fish net. It has three sides, with one side wider than the others. Fold the side that is widest and tie a knot at the fold. This will create a pocket and a better fit around the forehead. Place the knot in the center of the forehead. Tie the net in the back with the third end placed inside of the tie and the knot should be easy to remove. This net will hold the hair in place through the rinse of both the shampoo and the conditioner.

Use a generous amount of clarifying shampoo. It will clean deeper, quicker and more thoroughly. Do two or three applications of the shampoo, and allow the second and third one to sit for five full minutes. This will give the product a chance to dissolve the dirt, oils, and any build up on the hair.

Apply the shampoo using both hands, but if the hair is synthetic, be gentle. If you are very careful, you can massage it into a very thick lather. The thicker the lather the more ability the shampoo will have to break down any build up of oils and dirt and clean your hair and scalp. If it is your real hair, spend some time using your fingertips to massage your hair and scalp. If possible have the work done in the salon. If you must do the work at home, use your shower with the water as warm as you can stand it. When dealing with natural hair, the warmer the water, the better.

Conditioner Application for Natural Hair

If the conditioner is thick, dilute with water 50/50 in a spray bottle. It will make the conditioner easier to apply and easier to rinse. Spray the conditioner thoroughly on all of the hair. The conditioner should be left in the hair under a plastic cap for about thirty minutes. Use Hair Rebuilder cream conditioner, which is a treatment with every application. It re-builds badly damaged hair, it smells really good, and it works very well.

Be Natural but Relax

It is a woman's prerogative to change her mind anytime she wants and as often as she pleases. That's just one of the many things I love about a black woman. You go girl!

If after you have been wearing your hair natural for some time, you then wish to relax the hair, keep this in mind. To go from straight or chemically relaxed to natural, all of the hair that has been relaxed will eventually have to be removed. It is impossible for chemically relaxed hair to revert to natural. Don't let anyone tell you otherwise.

To go from natural back to straight is like taking candy from a baby. Spend about three weeks treating your hair with conditioners every four days. This equals seven treatments in twenty-one days. Allow four days between the last treatment and your chemical relaxer. This will prepare the hair for the chemical service. It is important to have the work done professionally, and make sure a *conditioning lye relaxer* is used.

Notice that I did not say *"No-Lye"* Relaxer.

A Conditioning Lye Relaxer, properly applied every time, including the retouch, is the very best way to chemically relax natural hair. It should always be followed with a quality conditioner plus a shampoo and a conditioner every five days like clockwork for the life of the hair. Allow no compromises and no exceptions. Make this a rule for your hair, follow it, and you will always have very beautiful hair, I promise. It's a natural thing, be natural, relax and enjoy your hair.

Wear a Hairstyle That Works Where You Work

If your hair doesn't look good to you, it probably doesn't look good to anyone else. I have seen some ugly hairdos in the work place. I have seen hair that looks like no one has touched it in months or longer, and I'm talking about black women. Some of them look like they just got up out of bed and went to work. Maybe someone is hoping for just the right time to talk to you about your hair.

The thing to consider is your work environment/setting, i.e. a bank, hotel lobby, a business office, an accounting firm or a law office or other setting. Consider the kinds of people you deal with each day. Consider your employer's overall image and dress code, even if you don't like what that is. If you are making a lot of money or have the potential or opportunity to get paid well, you may have to choose between the value of your job, and having your own way with your natural hairstyle. Someone once told me when you work for a man, work for him, and that means do what is required.

There is an easy way to work this out. Wear a hairstyle that works where you work, or go to the people you work for and ask questions. No matter what happens you will get an answer.

In certain work settings women of color often experience problems related to the acceptance of natural hairstyles, braids, extensions, and the like. This is the reason she is forever looking for a "wash and wear" hairdo, but there is no such thing. If you want beautiful hair, get to work. Remember, taking care of black hair is a full time job, and to grow and wear it natural is not necessarily easier, but it can become a lot easier if you do it right.

One thing is for sure, your intelligence, the ability to earn money for your employer and be paid what you are worth, are all separate issues. Expressing your individuality as a woman, black, attractive and wearing one of many natural hairstyles is also a separate issue. If you would change the way you feel and think about all of it, especially your hair, it could change the way everyone else feels. The way I see it, it's all-good.

The way you wear your hair in college or in a room filled with computers, or in a courtroom as an attorney, could all be perceived differently. It is a fact that people have hang-ups when it comes to hair, skin color, age and race, which seems to be a well-kept secret for people with such problems. Your problem may not be yours at all. It could be your attitude or their attitude or a number of other possibilities. I believe you can get around most. You know with certainty what you can and cannot do on your job. So it's simple. Do what you have to do. Wear your hair natural, only wear a hairstyle "that works" where you work. It will help if you keep the hair clean, healthy, and as pretty as it can be.

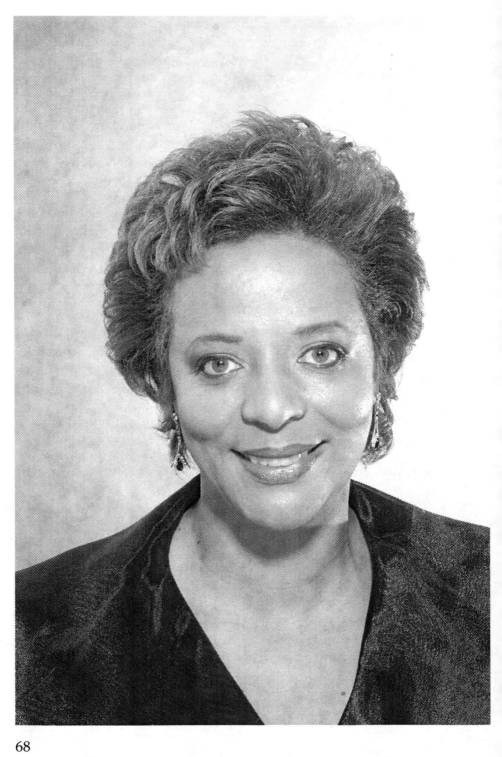

Chapter Six

Great Looking Hair Anywhere: How to Have Hair That Looks Great All the Time

If You Can't Stand the Heat, Get Out of the Kitchen

Like most black families, my family holds a family reunion celebration every year in a different location. The year that it was held near Orlando, Florida was one that I will long remember. I had always wanted to visit Florida, so my wife made all of the travel arrangements, and we took off. When we arrived in Florida, I became miserable, immediately. I do not like hot weather, and it was so hot in Florida, that I told my family, "I love you, and I love Orlando, but I'm never coming back here again!" It was just too hot and humid for me. So I did exactly like the old saying, "if you can't stand the heat, get out of the kitchen." I got out of Florida as fast as I could.

Hot Spots

If you live in one of the world's hot spots, you will find everything you will need to know to care for your hair in this chapter. If you intend to travel to one of these hot spots, stick this book in your suitcase so you can refer to it. You'll also need to know which products to use and what tools to carry along.

If you wear a relaxer or a curl, it is advisable to get a retouch before your trip. Make sure a conditioning lye relaxer is used. Purchase a moisturizing shampoo and a very high quality protein moisturizing conditioner. Be sure to take enough of a supply to last the entire trip.

The number one difficulty you will have to deal with where the weather is very hot is dry hair, and number two on the list is sweat from the humidity. Rainy, hot days will be "bad hair days" magnified to the 12th power. A lye relaxer, permanent haircolor, and the curl will all cause some dryness in your hair. If you are using no-lye relaxer in your hair, you can multiply the dryness by 1,000 percent.

You will want to have a large bottle of Humectress Moisturizing Conditioner from Nexxus Products on hand. It is the best for restoring much-needed moisture to hair that has been relaxed with a no-lye relaxer. All of the products recommended here are designed to impart moisture in differing degrees into the hair, which is exactly what your hair will need the most. This choice could also be the conditioner you have always used (your "regular" or "main"conditioner).

This is How It Works

Consider the following when selecting the right conditioner, shampoo, and other Hair Care Products:

- ❑ Your hair type
- ❑ Problems you may be experiencing at the moment
- ❑ Whether you have just had a new color job
- ❑ Whether you are wearing color and relaxer in your hair at the same time
- ❑ Whether your hair is dry, shedding, lifeless and so on.

It is important to remember that throughout your lifetime, your hair will change, and those changes will necessitate a change in your hair care product selection. Your hair may become weak and may start to break or shed for seemingly for no reason at all. It may change color overnight, after a swim, or simply because it's summertime. It may become very dry, oily, lifeless, frizzy or puffy without warning. Just the right shampoo and conditioner can change things for you tremendously. It can put new life back into your hair, or stop breakage in just twenty-four hours. Good conditioners do not dry out the hair, cause breakage, or weaken the hair in any way.

If you are vacationing, you will probably be in a hot spot no longer than one or two weeks, and you will probably want to do as little as possible to your hair.

Getting the Hair in Shape For Your Trip

❑ Four to six weeks before traveling, start your hair on a conditioning treatment regimen of every 4 or 5 days. Conditionin your hair is most important, whether traveling or at home.

❑ Use the same product you will be using on the trip.

❑ You may want to get a fresh haircut or a trim. This will give the hair balance and a neat appearance.

❑ If you intend to go swimming in the ocean, which is salt water, or in a pool, which contains chlorine, you must go to the shower immediately following your swim, before your hair has a chance to dry.

❑ Shampoo your hair three times. Deeply cleanse your hair of all the salt or chlorine.

❑ Condition the hair, and let the conditioner stay in five to ten minutes, then rinse very well.

❑ Spray in some setting lotion. This will help the hair to comb easier when wet.

❑ Dry the hair completely.

❑ After the hair is dry, mix a dime-size portion of Crème Press and a dime-size portion of PCA Moisture Retainer, and apply it to the hair.

❑ Use Crème Press daily in dime-size portions. This will help keep the hair from drying out.

When using quality Hair Care Products, know that they are designed to stop all of the breakage, and to make the hair stronger and more beautiful. Use regularly, and before you know it, you will have a head full of it. This works well for kids also.

Hot Spot Styling Tips: Wear cornrows, braids, pony-tails, updo's, or hats and scarves. You will need to carry along bobby pins, hairpins, butterfly clips, an assortment of accessory combs, a blow dryer with comb attachment, and one or two electric curling irons.

You will also need an adapter to plug things in. The electric outlets are different in various places.

If you live in a warm vacation location you are lucky. It really doesn't matter how your hair is cut, whether it is short, shoulder length or longer, you should follow the same shampoo and conditioning program. The secret to having beautiful healthy hair in a "hot spot," is in servicing the hair regularly, every four or five days, without exception. If you are wearing a conditioning lye relaxer and or permanent haircolor, shampooing and conditioning every four to five days is great; however, more often is better.

Is it Possible to Have Beautiful Hair Anywhere?

Yes! Yes! Yes! Having healthy hair is so simple. Yet, for most women of color, this presents a complicated and agonizing daily challenge. Is there any help in sight? Yes, Yes, Yes, so don't throw your hands in the air and act like you just don't care. Just read on because the answers are well within your reach.

Shine On, Shine On Beautiful Hair

Too much emphasis is placed on getting the hair to shine. The makers of Hair Care Products have been cashing in on this obsession for years, and what is so unbelievable, is that no matter what product you used to create the shine, it is but a passing fancy. The shine disappears almost as fast as it appears.

The natural appearance of black hair is one without shine. So why is so much money spent on making black hair shine? We believe that it makes our hair look healthy and less dry, which seems to imply that the hair is unhealthy. How do we fix it? We must adjust the way we look at our hair and except what we cannot change. People of other races secrete a lot more oil from the scalp. This is the reason they must shampoo and condition more often and on a regular basis. Black people secrete little or no oil.

Let's Get Physical

Let us assume that at this point you are following all of the recommendations and instructions outlined in this chapter. This may be the perfect time to get physical.

How Fat I Am—A True Story

When people used to comment on how fat I was, I would tell them that it was just more of me to love. February 14, 1994, I went into the hospital to have my stomach stapled, which consisted of making the stomach into a smaller pouch, in order to lose weight by not allowing me to over eat. This is something I will never do again, but it worked. I was 311 pounds at the time, I could not stay on my feet for very long, and I looked like a refrigerator. Following the surgery, I lost 125 pounds in about five months.

One day I was sitting waiting to see my doctor, and without thinking, I crossed my legs. It was then I realized that because my thighs had been so fat, I hadn't been able to cross my legs in years.

Let's Go Gyming— Hair, Sweat and You

It is a wonderful thing to be able to get up every day and go to the gym to work out. Exercising is good for your health and your hair. You are going to sweat a lot which will produce some salt in the moisture from the sweating, and the hair will get wet, or at least damp, in the process.

Stop believing the myth that you can't shampoo and condition your hair every day. The truth is you *can* shampoo and condition every day, *but* the key is to use quality Hair Care Products. Even shampooing and conditioning three or four times a week can be wonderful for your hair.

Perhaps your schedule is such that you have to go directly to work or school after your daily workout. In that case, shampooing and conditioning immediately after the workout is not possible. You can use a few style tips from the section entitled "Hot Spots." You must shampoo to clean your hair and free it of unwanted odors from sweat and salt. A conditioner should always follow the shampoo. So in the evening when you return home, if you worked out that day, exercise your hair's right to a shampoo and conditioner. If you believe that your edges, the hair around the face, will become nappy because of so many shampoos, consider the following.

Just because you had your hair relaxed a week or two earlier, don't think the hair will stop growing and stay straight forever. In fact, your hair is always growing, even while you're having it relaxed. You could possibly see new growth in as little as one or two days, and in two weeks you will definitely see new growth. To test this theory, look at the hair of someone who wears haircolor to cover gray. You will see new growth almost over night.

That's life and there is nothing we can do to stop hair from growing. Now isn't that a wonderful thought? The main concern should be keeping the hair on the head in a healthy, clean, and well-conditioned state. So let's get physical, and do the work that is required to have a marvelous head of hair. Then, let's go gyming to get the rest of you ready for your gorgeous new look.

Hair Care in Institutional Settings

Proper hair maintenance can be difficult in facilities where people are confined for extended periods of time. Such services are often limited or non-existent. Hospitals, nursing homes, and other long-term treatment facilities, are usually not equipped to provide the hair care services that women of color require.

Most hospital staff members have no idea how to care for the hair of black female patients. If the patient has family, this task is usually left up to them. Sometimes the family will supply a wig, or a family member or friend will come in a few times a week to take care of the patient's hair.

Sometimes the family will purchase products, and instruct staff on their proper usage. If there is a black attendant or staff member, they may offer to assist with the patient's hair care. If patients are alert and ambulatory, they may do each other's hair.

The Truth About Heat and Chemicals

I visited a very popular salon in New York City and spent a day observing a master designer at work. He had four assistants, and all he did was roller sets that started at $50.00 and went up from there.

He believes that heat from hot irons, blow-dryers, hot combs and heated rollers is bad for black hair, and he advises his clients against their use.

Let's Agree to Disagree

If you have lost much of your own hair, you may be nodding your head in agreement with this master hair designer's point of view. If so, you are both right and wrong. Keep reading and I'll explain.

Styling this way is wonderful and very healthy for your hair, but it does not mean that using hot irons, blow-dryers, chemicals and such can't also be healthy for your hair, or in some cases, better for your hair. Sometimes "less is more," but when styling roller sets, the finished look won't last long enough for you to get out the chair and pay your bill. If you don't roll your hair, the next morning you will wake up with straight hair that has no curl, no shape or style, and no body because nothing was applied to the hair to help it hold the curls or any wave pattern.

When the hair is chemically relaxed, all of its ability to curl and hold a curl is gone forever. Sometimes fifteen or twenty percent of the natural curl is left in the hair, and this is good, but hair that has been relaxed this way still will not hold curls. What do you do? You break out those hot curling irons you were told to stay away from, and you get busy hot curling your hair.

There Are Professionals In Every Category of This Business

When I am styling hair, I use chemical relaxers, a blow-dryer and my hot irons all the time. The irons I use are Marcel irons, which require maximum heat to do the job well.

- ❑ The finished look is always soft, always has sheen, and the curls last three to five days or longer.
- ❑ The hair is never dry.
- ❑ The hair is never damaged and never falls out.

How is all of this possible? Product knowledge. Understanding how to use the products and which ones to use to protect the hair from the heat makes it possible. In these pages you can learn all of my secrets too. Most of you are having problems because you don't put anything on the hair to protect it from the heat. You are using the wrong kinds of relaxers, shampoos, conditioners and everything else. The hair gets very dry, and you lose a lot of hair. Let's face it, everyone is not going to stop using hair dryers, curling irons, relaxers, no-lye relaxers, or other wise.

So what does this have to do with avoiding heat and chemicals? It is neither the heat nor the chemicals that are destructive to your hair, actually it is the *person* applying the heat and the chemicals. Put the book down, and go to the closest mirror. Who do you see?

The person you see is public enemy number one. Now, sing these words out loud, "He's talk'n 'bout the girl in the mirror. She's the only one who can make that change." You must change everything you have been doing to your hair—starting NOW.

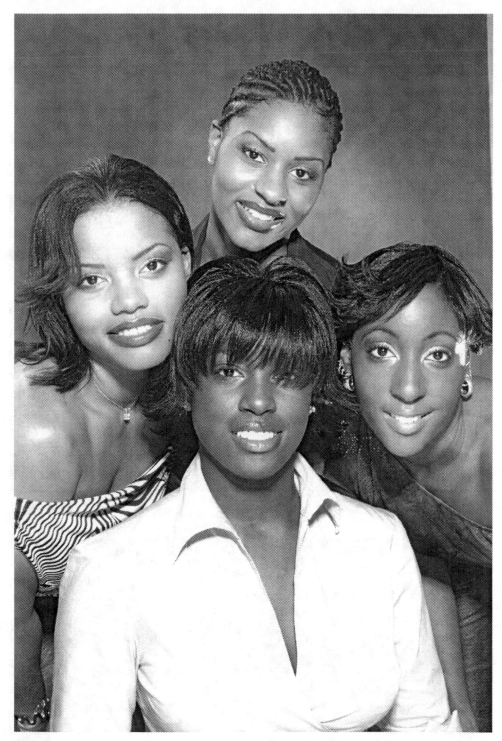

Shamboosie's

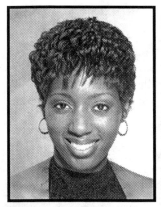 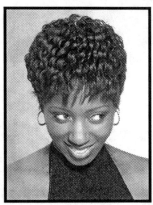 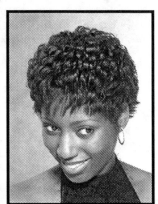

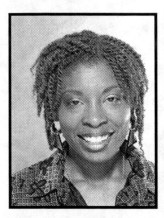 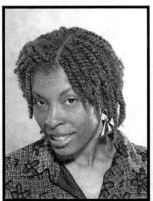 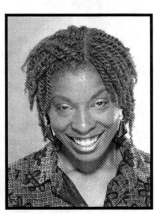

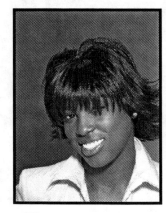 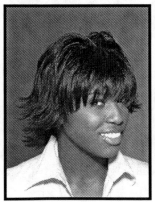 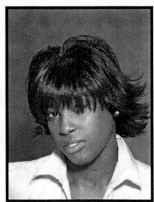

Style Gallery

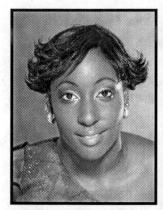 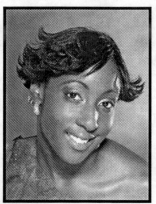 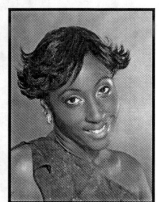

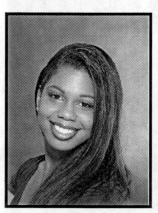 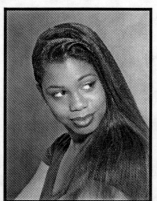 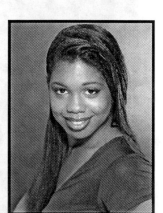

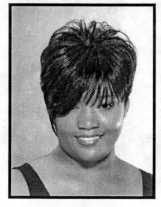 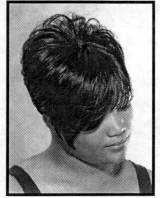 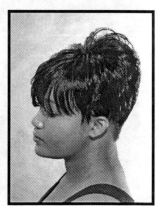

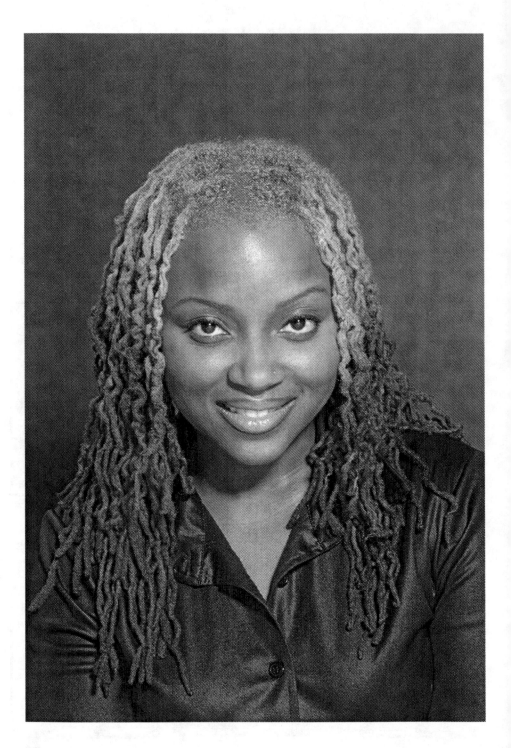

Chapter Seven

The Color of Hair

The Coloring Book: Understanding Haircolor

To really understand the coloring process you must first understand natural haircolor and how it came to be. First of all every person is special, and one of a kind. No two people have the same eyes or fingerprints, and the most amazing thing is no two have the same natural haircolor. Most black people think their hair is black, but the fact is our hair is many dark shades of brown, and never black. Actually, there are as many different natural haircolors as there are people. The understanding of these natural shades is the science that makes the choices and decisions about coloring the hair possible.

A Closer Look at Hair

We have said that hair is a slender, thin, thread-like fiber composed mostly of different types of protein, about 98%, which is also referred to as keratin. The bottom end of the appendage or hair strand is where the hair receives its nourishment. The size and shape of the hair will be determined by the size and shape of the follicle. If the opening of the follicle is round, the hair will be straight. If it is flat, the hair will be curly or kinky, and if oval in shape, the hair will be wavy.

There Are Three Layers—Cuticle, Cortex & Medulla

The *Cuticle* or the protective layer. When chemicals are applied the hair, they raise the cuticles, allowing them access into the cortex. The *Cortex*, the second layer is where the action is because everything you put on or into your hair, enters through the cuticles, and change everything about the hair in the cortex. This includes shampoos, conditioners, permanent haircolors and the greatest changes occur with the application of the chemical relaxer.

The *Cortex* is where many of the bonds are located, and where Ammonia/Peroxide-based haircolors, chemical relaxers, perms, conditioners and other chemicals will cause a more permanent change in the texture, pigmentation, and wave pattern of the hair. In most cases, the changes occur in the hair from the inside out, and many of those changes are permanent.

When **The Rules** are broken, the cuticle will also suffer. A healthy, very well-conditioned cuticle layer is the only way to protect the cortex layer. When the cuticle is badly damaged, the cortex is exposed, and the hair becomes weak, lifeless, and almost impossible to manage. With time, it will start to look like anything but hair, and fall out.

When you understand the effects every chemical and every product has on the hair, you will be able to use this information to avoid those things, the wrong types of products, and improper application techniques that have been causing all of the problems.

The *Medulla* you don't have, but one or more can be found in other hair types. The more Medullas, the softer and more porous the hair is because the Medulla is somewhat mushy or spongy in texture. The term porous means the hair's ability to absorb moisture. This makes the hair really susceptible to possible damage.

More Natural Properties of Hair

Melanin is the natural color Mother Nature puts in hair. The amount, type and density of melanin in hair, determines its natural color. There are three types, Eumelanin that is synonymous to the dark pigmentation in black, medium brown and lighter colors of blonde hair. Pheomelanin gives the hair most of its rose colors, orange, and gold, and a mixture Eumelanin and Pheomelanin called Mixed Melanin, concerns itself with the golden brown tones in the hair. Understanding the natural pigmentation of the hair will help you to come up with the perfect colors and shades every time. The natural degrees of lightness and darkness in the color of the hair must always be taken into account. Don't panic, the makers of haircolor have made all of this easier for you, and have worked out most of it in their formulas. Just follow a few simple rules, and all should be fine.

 A Color Tip: Anytime chemicals are misused, the chance of losing hair is almost 100% guaranteed. The chance of saving the hair is slim, but possible, because once these chemicals are put in the hair, the changes they make in the structure and texture of the hair cannot be reversed. The hair will get weaker and weaker with time, becoming more and more difficult to manage. This is the reason education is so very important. You must know exactly what you are doing to the hair and how it will affect the hair at all times.

A New Permanent Coloring Solution for Chemically Relaxed Hair

All of the years that I have been a part of the hair & beauty industry I have wondered when someone, would bridge the gap between permanent haircolor and the chemical relaxer. Such an inventor would have to formulate both the relaxer and the permanent haircolor. Then both products would have to share many of the same properties in order to work well together. The creator of such a product would also have to research and eliminate the hindrances and the concerns that have prevented the use of permanent haircolor on chemically treated hair.

Dispelling the Myths

Before we continue this dialog on haircolor, you should know that Shamboosie recommends that you always consult with a professional colorist to have all of your color work done.

Now, just what does all of this mean? In most salons, the very idea of applying permanent haircolor to chemically relaxed hair is strictly taboo. It has been that way longer than I have been a part of the industry. In fact, a few other terms come to mind like "forbidden," a "hands-off approach," "impermissible," "banned," "prohibited," "disallowed," and the very idea seems to scared the heck out of just about everyone, clients and professionals alike.

Most of the fear does not come from personal experiences with applying permanent haircolor to chemically relaxed hair, but instead it comes from myths, stories, and even lies that have been passed around from home to home, from salon to salon, from hairdresser to hairdresser, and even from hair school to hair school. Yes, a lot of black people have had some very bad experiences with permanent haircolor. All of it comes from mistakes made due to a lack of knowledge by people who have been coloring their hair at home, and by hair professionals, that simply don't understand the theory and art of coloring hair.

The Coloring Book was written to show all of the areas to stay away from, the numerous coloring possibilities, shades and techniques, and all of the things you need to know to be successful in your quest to wear your hair any color you like.

So What's The Big Deal About Haircolor & Chemically Relaxed Hair?

If you were to ask this question of most hair care professionals of black hair, most would say "permanent coloring, in chemically relaxed hair will cause the hair to fall out." What they are really saying is they don't know how to do it and still keep the hair from falling out. So the whole problem is a lack of knowledge. But all of the answers, all of the know-how is available, and it has always been available. Many hair care professionals and laypersons alike are not aware of the reasons why permanent haircolor renders the hair so fragile, porous, soft, and dry. The thought of applying relaxer to hair in such a condition is alarming, even terrifying.

The Cause of These Problems

Permanent haircolor is formulated two ways, as an *oxidizing* color, which means that when left in the open air the chemicals are activated starting the developing process of the color, and a *non-oxidizing* chemical, which has no lifting properties. One of the ingredients in an oxidizing permanent haircolor formula is **ammonia**. When ammonia is mixed with peroxide, it forms a third chemical that enables the formula to lift, or change the natural color of your hair, while at the same time it is depositing a newly-developed synthetic color. There is no ammonia, therefore no lifting ability, with the non-oxidizing haircolor. To make a permanent coloring product for chemically relaxed hair, the chemist has found a way around the use of ammonia in permanent haircolor, that still gives it the ability to lift natural haircolor and deposit synthetic color. The problem is that most of us have been using an oxidizing formula.

Ammonia, when mixed with peroxide, lifts or removes color, and it causes the hair to swell during the process. This swelling remains a part of the hair for the life of that hair. This is an extreme change in the texture of the hair causing it to become softer, spongy, porous, and more absorbent. The problem is that ammonia also causes the hair to become dryer, weaker, more fragile and susceptible to breakage.

Therein lies one of the primary problems with permanent haircolor and chemically relaxed hair. Hair in this condition will continue to digress with time, if the hair is not properly cared for and conditioned on a regular basis. Even then the hair will still be quite delicate. So your choice for permanently coloring your hair is one *without* ammonia. The key to proper care is a combination of just the right conditioners for each individual head of hair, because they are all different.

The thing that is so frightening, and is also obscured by a lack of knowledge is the proper process of application, when it's time to chemically relax or retouch the new growth. It is believed that the hair will not be strong enough to handle the chemical relaxer, and there is reason for concern. It is also thought that the relaxer will eat through the hair shaft, literally dissolve the hair or damage it to such a degree that the hair will come out. This too is highly possible, and it has happened many times to many people.

These are the major concerns of most black hairstylists in the business, but this doesn't mean that it has to happen, or that it is supposed to happen. In fact, it is not supposed to happen, and it will not happen if all of the proper procedures are learned and followed with every application of permanent haircolor and the chemical relaxer. The key here is to stay within the boundaries and the laws and theory of cosmetology.

Colors—But a Passing Fancy

Temporary Colors are just that, temporary. Once they are applied you can be sure they are short-lived. There is no heat involved, and they are the perfect colors to wear for a weekend, and are usually washed out with the first shampoo. The best results are derived from applying the product to wet hair, before the application of the conditioner. Rinse with cool water until the water runs clear and do not shampoo. Temporary colors have no lifting properties, no chemicals, and will only coat the hair shaft. Reds and black are the most noticeable when they are applied. These colors can also be applied the same day as a chemical relaxer.

Semi-permanent Colors are temporary colors that are placed under a plastic cap, then under a warm dryer for 30 minutes. The heat causes the color to penetrate, and stay on the hair a bit longer, 1 or 2 shampoos. Again, these colors will only deposit, and they have no developer or ammonia in the formula.

Long Lasting Semi-permanent Colors involve a low volume developer of 10 or less. It is the 10-volume developer that causes these colors to last much longer. It will also allow you to change or lift your natural haircolor just enough to notice. Mix the 2 ounces of 10-volume developer to a color 1 or 2-levels lighter than your natural level and process for 20 to 30 minutes. Rinse, shampoo once, condition, and style.

Memorize the Basic Rules

The basic rules for using haircolor and other chemicals will never change, and will come into play every time you color, relax, perm, shampoo or condition your hair. Each chemical product will have its own set of rules. Learning all of them, which is really very easy to do, will be the secret to your success. This book will provide all of the rules and solutions to your haircolor and hair care problems.

1. When most people do the relaxer retouch, they apply the chemical far past the *line of demarcation* (where the color-treated hair connects with the new growth,) by combing it through the hair. This is the way many people are used to applying relaxer, and it is indeed the wrong way, even when color-treated hair is not involved. **The Rule**—the chemical must be applied to the new growth only, and maintained in that area.

    I assure you that the relaxer creme will move on its own, slightly past the line of demarcation, especially when the hair is short, but the problem is in combing the chemical through the hair. Remember the relaxer will do all of its own work and will complete its job in about 13 to 15 minutes. See The System.

2. Another reason is that the chemical relaxer is probably the wrong strength. **The Rule**—it must always be a mild relaxer (no exceptions).

3. No precaution has been taken to protect the hair. **The Rule**—The color treated hair must always be coated with setting gel or crème conditioner to protect the hair from the relaxer, before the chemical is applied.

4. Never underestimate the power of a good conditioner. **The Rule**—The proper deep conditioning treatment must always follow the retouch relaxer and the retouch of the permanent haircolor.

5. **The Rule**—Always complete the relaxer retouch before the permanent color retouch, and relax the virgin hair (hair that has never been colored) before coloring altogether. The reason is obvious; the relaxer is the stronger of the two.

6. Some people have badly damaged hair or very weak hair. Others have hair that is under-conditioned. If permanent haircolor is added to the mix, hair in this condition will be compromised in the process. **The Rule**—Never apply permanent haircolor in this case.

7. **The Rule**—You must know the outcome before starting the coloring process. This is true in applying both the relaxer and the haircolor. Most people will apply color and hope that it all will come out okay—it doesn't, ever. To be certain of the outcome, you will have to know how many levels the developer mixed with ammonia and the color will lift the natural haircolor when the developer is 10, 20, or 30 volume. They all will be different, have a different effect on the hair, and even the shade of the color will affect the outcome.

9. **The Rule**—The longer a peroxide base haircolor stays on the hair, the greater its effect on the hair, or the more it will change the texture of that hair.

10. It is amazing how many people are using the wrong volume of developer for the job. Peroxide comes in different volumes for a reason, and the idea that one is as good as the other is the farthest thing from the truth. **The Rule**—40 volume developer should never be a part of the equation.

11. **The Rule**—You must determine the level of the natural haircolor. There are only 10 possible levels, which will be covered later. Everyone's natural haircolor will fall within one of the 10 levels. Knowing the level of the natural haircolor will help you determine how many levels and shades the hair will

have to be changed to reach your desired shade destination. It will aid you in determining the exact haircolor and developer to use to achieve the end result.

12. **The Rule**—You must determine the level and shade you want the hair to be in the end result. This will be easier than you think because you don't have to be exact. Actually, there is no way you can be exact. There are so many different colors and shades to choose from that are very close to each other and to your desired shade. In this case, close counts, and besides, no two applications, even with the same formula, will turn out the same every time. The reason is because the final result will always be a product of the color to be applied to the hair and the colors that are already in the hair. The final shade and color could turn out lighter, darker, or anything in between. So close is good enough.

13. You must decide on the method of application. **The Rule**—The hair will always dictate. This one is simple you only have to decide if you want to go up in color, down in color, or remain right where you are and blend in. Then you must decide if it is to be a virgin application or a retouch application. Knowing this will aid you in deciding the exact formula to be mixed for the job?

New Technology

This term is so appropriate in today's world of computers and other digital gadgets. The term is also appropriate as it relates to hair care. The one thing we must always look for in this beauty business is improvements in product for chemically treated hair. There are new developments made all the time. Upgrades form the New Technology on permanent haircolor, and conditioners are better than ever. Shampoo formulas are now specialized, oils are lighter, hairdressing really does make the hair prettier. Hairsprays made especially for black hair give a better hold without drying the hair out. Gels are less flaky, less drying, and most importantly conditioning relaxers are infused with more high quality conditioning properties than ever before, and they do a better job than ever.

Back to The Future

It seems like everyone in the beauty business is still living in the past, using the same old techniques, and Hair Care Products, and servicing clients with the same old 1500 hours of basic education, with few, if any, upgrades. I am sure there are hairdressers out there somewhere trying to improve on their knowledge and skills, and a few that are aware of some of the New Technology in the industry.

Haircolor manufacturers are now starting to pursue New Technology for designing permanent haircolor that can be applied to hair that has been chemically relaxed, with a safer outcome.

I have personally been involved with the test marketing of two new formulas, and find them to be exquisite. It is the most exiting news I have heard in 20 years— Clairol's Textures & Tones Conditioning haircolor and what Clairol calls "a gentle art," Beautiful Collection Gentle Crème Permanent Color. The possibilities are creatively exhilarating.

No Ammonia Means a Lot Less Damage

Ammonia in permanent haircolor causes the hair to become very dry and porous after the color service. It is the one ingredient in permanent haircolor that does the most damage. Now this will surprise you, most people in the hair care profession are not aware of this fact. It is also the reason most people who style chemically-treated hair prefer not to permanently color hair. The removal or reduction of ammonia has made permanent haircolor for chemically-relaxed hair much safer. It is also better for everyone else's hair. In addition, an assortment of conditioning ingredients such as aloe vera, moisturizers, vitamins, jojoba, protein, and many other oils have been added to help strengthen and keep the hair moist and soft after the color service. These products have a *non-drying* effect on the hair. So the types of permanent haircolor you want to shop for are colors that do not contain ammonia, but do contain volumes of quality conditioners.

Women of color can now chemically relax and permanently color their hair, while at the same time leaving the hair in a much healthier condition than ever before.

The Rule—Remember to allow at least seven full days, and one shampoo and a conditioning treatment between the two processes.

 A Color Tip: Haircolor, Bleach, and Thio, the curly perm, all will cause the three layers to become very soft and porous especially, the cuticle layer. Depending on the degree of alteration, repair could be possible. However, the repair will be temporary but repeatable with little damage, and not possible at all if the damage is severe. Education is the key to avoiding the problems. In every case use a very good protein/moisturizing conditioner.

Product Knowledge

Clairol's Textures & Tones Conditioning haircolor is a fresh new approach to haircolor especially formulated for women of color, and for chemically relaxed hair. This means beautiful, permanent haircolor, with no worry when it's time for a retouch of the chemical relaxer is finally possible! It is important to follow the proper relaxer application techniques that are found in the System #1, to insure the safest and healthiest end result.

It is formulated with Elasticom, a unique moisturizing complex with panthenol, Brazil nut oil, wheat protein and many other special conditioners. These innovative conditioning properties leave the hair moisturized, soft, silky, and healthy-looking with every application.

Textures & Tones Haircolor is the first ammonia-free permanent haircolor enriched with Elasticom, that protects relaxed hair from damage during the coloring process. It provides permanent, moisture-drenched color, and 100% gray coverage every time. **Remember, it is the ammonia in haircolor that has been causing many of the problems with permanent haircolor and chemically relaxed hair.**

Textures & Tones

This is the only complete, dual system of permanent haircolor and conditioning cream relaxers of its kind in the marketplace. *Textures & Tones* is an innovative line of incredible Hair Care Products especially designed for women of color. I personally recommend the use of this complete system.

The Haircoloring System

1. Should be used with a developer

2. Imparts ultimate moisture, elasticity and shine

3. Covers gray 100% and will highlight selected strands of hair.

4. It is available in 7 shades.

The Hair Care System

1. One-Minute Reconstructive Conditioner (This is a wonderful treatment. I strongly recommend it.)

2. Neutralizing Shampoo

3. Ultra-Moisture Shampoo

4. Balanced Crème Hairdress

5. Light Moisturizing Oil Shiner & Styling Gel

The Conditioning Crème Lye Relaxer

1. Provides moisture and protection during the straightening process.

2. Contains Elasticom, a unique moisturizing complex that infuses hair with nutrients.

3. Provides conditioning that you can feel, even after rinsing.

4. Removes natural curl with ease.

5. Texturizes the hair by removing a small amount of its natural curl.

Most renowned for fortifying ingredients that leave hair soft, silky, healthy, manageable and strong, Textures & Tones moisturizing, conditioning and protective properties have allowed it to become one of the top choices available for women of color. It's beauty without compromise. I personally recommend it.

Clairol Professional features many formulas suitable and safe for use on chemically treated hair. In addition, they provide a conditioner base with each application of the highest quality.

General Usage
▼ To match or deepen color - Use 10-volume
▼ To cover gray hair - Use 20-volume
▼ To lighten natural haircolor – Use 30-volume

Mixing
▼ Mix 2 oz of the product with 2 oz of developer
▼ For bowl and brush application, mix with Pure White cream developer.

The Greatest Upgrade of the Decade

Removing the ammonia from permanent haircolor entirely changes the whole picture. The integrity of the hair, the very texture, is only slightly changed, and that slight change is a beautiful new haircolor. The swelling of the hair, dryness, and the porosity are all gone forever. The unique moisturizing complex Elasticom, with panthenol, Brazil nut oil, wheat protein and other special conditioners are the essential additions that have brought about this revolutionary resolve to bridge the gap between permanent haircolor and the conditioning lye relaxer in black hair. Elasticom strengthens the hair shaft internally and externally, improving and protecting the hair's resistance to breakage. So now you can permanently color your hair and relax, just not on the same day.

Beautiful Collection Gentle Crème Permanent Colors— another permanent haircolor designed for relaxed hair. This one is truly a gentle art, meaning that it lifts your natural haircolor gently. It lightens and darkens your hair gently. It conditions as it colors and is enriched with Vitamin E, Aloe Vera, and Jojoba Oil to protect, moisturize and add shine, leaving the hair rich in color, healthier and stronger after each application.

Plus they can change your natural color or cover up to 100% gray. There are eight beautiful shades.

Temporary & Semi-Permanent Colors

Clairol's Jazzing offers translucent shades that will spice up haircolor with temporary or semi-permanent results. Because these colors are temporary, they will only coat the hair shaft. If you were to pre-lighten your hair before applying Jazzing, the deposit would be greater and longer lasting. Pre-lightening will cause the hair to become porous, which means the hair will absorb more of the applied color. The same can be said for all temporary and semi-permanent haircolor. The difference is that Jazzing actually leaves the hair healthier, with shine, and conditions very well. Jazzing has no ammonia and no peroxide.

Each of the 19 dramatic shades *deposits only*, and adds sizzling, vibrant color, soft, subtle shades, that add richness and depth to natural haircolor. It restores luster, color, and conditions immediately after a chemical relaxer. Jazzing blends gray, enhances, matches, or brightens haircolor. It provides temporary results without heat, and semi-permanent results with heat.

A Whiter Shade of Pale

"Mary had a little girl whose hair was white as snow, and every time she colored her hair, the white hair continued to grow." This is a true story of a lovely 16-year-old black girl who had naturally white hair, which she had been coloring most of her young life. Like many, she used "jet-black" permanent haircolor every three or four weeks in addition to chemically relaxing her hair. With many of my clients I have to color and relax their hair also. So you see it is possible. Hair usually turns gray with age, but when it happens to a young person, it can become a rather trying experience, to say the least. It is just one of the many mysteries of life.

Have you ever heard the phrase, "men don't like roots"? What it means is after having their hair colored, they don't like to see the return of gray hair at the scalp, which is new growth. Believe me when I tell you that women don't like roots either.

This lovely 16-year-old girl is probably about 25 years old now, and chances are she is still spending a lot of money on hair coloring. The good news is that she, and others like her, can now wear their hair any color they choose, and there are lots of colors to choose from. Many entertainers in today's pop culture are wearing a rainbow of colors, which has become commonplace.

Gray Hair

I have seen many lovely shades of gray, white, and silver hair. Some shades of gray can be so beautiful it would be shameful to cover them or color them. Gray can be quite beautiful on some people, especially when it happens to someone in their early thirty's. Whether you desire to cover, color, blend, or flaunt your gray hair, I hope the information and advice stated here will help you do it beautifully.

The Quantity of Gray Dictates

Coloring, blending, or enhancing gray hair can be very difficult or very easy, depending upon how much you know about gray hair. In the hair care business, we measure the percentage of gray hair as *less than 25 percent, more than 25 percent, 50 percent and above,* and *100 percent*. The method of coloring or covering gray is determined by the percentage of gray. If you have less than 25 percent gray, and it is scattered equally throughout the head, a semi-permanent color will work in most cases, and when properly applied will last about 1 to 3 weeks or 2 shampoos, which ever comes first. Many black hair salons use a temporary color for this purpose, and many times it will last only about one week, if you are lucky. There are improvements in semi-permanent haircolors that have greater staining, and conditioning properties.

A Perfect Solution

The Rule—With chemically relaxed hair only, to go darker in color and shade, to remain the same color and shade or to just blend the gray, you will seldom need more than a 10-volume developer to complete the job. The reason? No lifting of any color is involved, only deposit, and a very low volume developer will allow this with no problem.

Relax & Permanently Color the Same Day— Yes It Can Be Done

Shamboosie's Solution: If your gray hair is less than 30%, and you want to cover it well, here is one solution that will work every time. It is permanent haircolor, but it works like a semi-permanent, and will last 4-6 weeks or longer. This formula is also safe to use on relaxed hair, and *can be applied on the same day as the relaxer*. Keep in mind that this formula should only be used to cover or blend gray hair when it is *less than 30 percent*, or if you want to go *one shade darker* than your natural haircolor. The actual shade or color of the your hair, and the product doesn't matter.

This is How We Do It

- ❑ Mix 1 ounce of the color of your choice with 1 ounce of 10 or 20-volume developer and 3 ounces of regular shampoo.
- ❑ Shake gently but well.
- ❑ Allow the bottle to sit with the top off until the formula develops and changes color. This will happen in about 5 minutes, so keep an eye on the formula. It must be applied a soon as it develops.
- ❑ Apply the formula to all of the hair or the area you wish to cover.
- ❑ Set a timer for ten minutes, and *do not* exceed the time limit.
- ❑ Rinse well, shampoo once, condition the hair, and style as usual.

❏ The next application should be a semi-permanent color of the same shade.

❏ Then alternate ever 3-4 weeks as needed.

The Secret to this Formula

The secret is the 3 ounces of shampoo. It weakens the 1-ounce of 10 or 20 volume developer considerably, but allows just enough strength to develop the color while it is still in the bottle. This formula in its weakened state will only allow the color to *stain* the hair in the 10-minute time limit, making it safe for use on freshly relaxed hair.

Twenty-five to 35 percent of gray hair will always need a long lasting semi-permanent haircolor, and this is a solution. This will mean at least a 10 or 20-volume developer will be added to the mix, which will cause haircolor to penetrate deeper into the cortex layer of the hair. The color will last about four weeks, perhaps five or six if you are really lucky. When the percentage of gray is between 35 percent or 100 percent, a permanent haircolor with 20-volume developer, and with no shampoo added, works best. A retouch on the color should take place in about four to six weeks, but only because of the new-growth, and only after the relaxer retouch.

What About That Big White Spot in Front?

Occasionally, there is a patch of gray in the front area with all of the rest of the hair on the head about 20 to 25 percent gray. To cover this type of gray patch, mix 1 ounce of color with 1 ounce of 20-volume developer, and apply it to this area *only*. The higher the percentage of gray, the more the type of haircolor you choose will have to have the ability to cover or color your gray. This is the reason *temporary* and *semi-permanent* haircolor will not cover the gray hair very well when the percentage of gray is greater than 20 percent. How then can one use *permanent* haircolor safely while at the same time having the hair chemically relaxed?

You no longer have to settle for "basic black." One can wear any color or any mixture of colors. Gray hair has no pigmentation or color, and can be very resistant and very difficult to color. This is because the color solution will not properly penetrate the hair shaft. If the hair is also coarse, it can add to the problem of coloring the hair. If this is the case, you may want to: pre-soften the hair with two ounces of a neutral or a clear color, mixed with two ounces of 20-volume developer.

❑ Process for 20 minutes.

❑ Apply the desired color formula also mixed with a 20-volume developer.

❑ Process for an additional 25 minutes, but do not exceed 45 minutes total.

❑ Check the hair after ten minutes, then every five minutes until completion.

❑ Remove the formula as soon as the hair is ready.

An Alternative for "Hard-to-Color" Gray Hair

1. Increase the developer to 30-volume.

2. Use a shade one level lighter than the color you want your hair to be.

3. Process up to 45 minutes.

4. Check after 20 minutes, then every five minutes.

5. Remove the formula as soon as the hair is ready, which may be less than the full 45 minute allotted time.

How Can You Tell if The Hair is Ready?

Pick up a section of the hair and use a wet towel to remove as much product from the hair as possible. You should be able to see the new color and shade. Keep in mind that because the hair is wet, it will appear to be darker in color. The true color will only appear after the hair has been dried. If you find that the hair is not ready, re-apply the formula and check a different section in 5 or 10 minutes.

Keep the Details Handy

Use only the amount of time you need, which could be less, but never greater than 45 minutes. This is when you are using a permanent haircolor. With *temporary* and *semi-permanent* haircolor, the longer the color stays on the hair the better. Use the full amount of time allowed. Remember, there is an assortment of color formulas available that can also be mixed to formulate something quite lovely and special for your hair. Be sure to keep a detailed record for future reference. Even if the work is performed in the salon, you should keep a copy of the record, which should include:

▼ The color formulation

▼ The name brand and color name or number

▼ Strength of the developer and type—crème, or liquid

▼ The exact method of application

▼ The exact amount of each ingredient added to the formula

▼ The exact amount of time the color was left on the hair

▼ Type of shampoo and conditioner (choose one for color-treated hair)

▼ The number of weeks between applications (be consistent)

▼ If possible, record the temperature of the room. (warm-cool-cold)

Learn to love your hair as much as you love yourself. Then you will do what is needed to grow it beautiful and to keep it that way. Good luck, and color with care.

You'll Wonder Where the Yellow Went

You can be sure that when the hair is pretty and white or gray, it will get dirty and turn yellow. Remember, violet cancels yellow. I can remember when I was a young boy, seeing the little old ladies in church with hair the color of blue-violet. This was the result of misuse of a shampoo product designed to remove the yellow from their gray hair. There are many such products on the market. When using this kind of yellow removing product, make sure to work *all* of the applied product into a thick lather. The yellow neutralizing shampoo product is violet in color. If any of the product is left on the hair without being worked into a lather, the gray or white hair will be left with a blue-violet color, which is the color of the product. Once it dries in the hair, removing this unwanted color becomes very difficult.

Yellow in gray hair can be caused by a build-up of styling aids like hairsprays, spritz, oils or setting gels. Yellow can also be the result of dirty hot curling irons, medication, or lack of proper shampoo and conditioning.

 A Color Tip: Choose a clear or neutral haircolor. Mix with two ounces of 10-volume developer, and apply to dry hair. Process for 25 minutes, rinse, shampoo, condition, and style as usual. There are many ways to neutralize yellow when the hair has more yellow than you desire, be it in gray hair or even when coloring the hair. There are many products on the market that are made especially for removing yellow. As with every Hair Care Product, read all of the manufacturer's suggestions and directions carefully and completely before you buy them, and before you apply them.

The pH Scale

PH is the symbol for *Potential Hydrogen Concentration*, which is the degree of acidity or alkalinity in a product. It is not important that you know the meaning of these terms. Just know that everything we use *on* or *in* our hair is a chemical, including water. In fact, water is the one constant in most Hair Care Products, except those that are in dry form. The acidity or alkalinity of each is measured on what is called a *pH scale*.

The pH scale goes from 0 to 14, with 7 being the balancing point. Everything to the left of 7 is acid, and everything to the right of 7 is alkaline. The closer a product is to 7, whether acid or alkaline, the milder and less harsh the product. Curls, haircolor, and relaxers all fall on the alkaline side of the pH scale. All of these products cause the hair to swell and leave the hair soft and porous. On the other hand, neutralizers, some conditioners, and peroxide all harden the hair and fall on the acid side of the scale.

The closer a product is to 1 on the acid side, the stronger it is, and the closer a product is to 14 on the alkaline side, the stronger it is. The difference in the types of shampoos, and the factor to be considered when selecting a shampoo, is whether it is pH balanced, which means it is not a harsh product. Its detergent is mild and gentle, which makes it perfect for use on chemically-treated hair. The one you should use is about 4.5 on the pH scale.

List of pH values

Color rinses	2.5
Vinegar	2.7
Neutralizers	3.0
Hair	4.5 to 5.0
Hydrogen peroxide	4.0
Skin	4.5 to 6.0
Shampoo (for your hair type)	4.0 to 4.5
Water	7
Blood	7.5

Stronger shampoos	7.0 to 10.0
Water softeners	10.5
Hair straighteners	11.0
Ammonia	11.8
Bleach or lightners	12.0 to 14
Lye relaxers	14.0
No-lye relaxer	14.0 to around 18.0, which is off the scale

When we chemically relax hair with a **conditioning lye relaxer**, it shoots up very high on the pH scale. When the hair is neutralized, which is done with a neutralizer in shampoo form, it will bring the pH of the hair back down, and normalize the hair around 8.5 and 7.0 in two to three days after the service. The hair needs the time to return to 7.0, and it will need a very good shampoo and conditioner before permanently coloring the hair, about a week later.

Imagine The Perfect Conditioning Situation

You have just had your hair relaxed with this conditioning crème relaxer, which has conditioned your hair with a unique moisturizing complex, Elasticom. The neutralizing shampoo continues the conditioning process because it also contains Elasticom. After every relaxer retouch, you must apply a conditioning treatment. **The One Minute Reconstructive Conditioner** really works in only one minute, and that's quick. I have repeatedly talked about quality Hair Care Product. Elasticom penetrates the hair quickly, it fortifies, which means it strengthens or invigorates the hair.

It nourishes, protects, and imparts a silky, healthy, reflective sheen without leaving a greasy, heavy feeling to the hair. One week later you return to have some color work done. The new Textures & Tones Red Hot Red, Burgundy Blaze, Ruby Rage and Flaming Desire, are all red, permanent, and beautiful shades on black ladies. They contain *no ammonia* and the conditioning complex, Elasticom. I personally went out and checked the stores to see if any other makers of permanent haircolor have anything close to this product line, designed especially for women of color. There are none, and this is the reason I recommend this particular line.

Your Hair's Pigmentation

Hair is made mostly of protein also known as *keratin*. When hair is in its most healthy condition, it reflects light, causing the hair to shine. The pigmentation, which is actually the color in the hair, remains your natural haircolor until something is done to alter the hair's natural color. Remember that white or gray hair has no color. The art of coloring the hair involves artificially changing the natural haircolor or pigmentation.

There are a few important things to keep in mind when doing haircolor at home: such as the *warmth* or *coolness* of a color, tonality, and most importantly, the contributing pigments, which are colors that are hidden in the hair's natural pigmentation and are revealed only when removing the hair's natural color with a bleach. These contributing colors will cause the majority of the problems you will have when permanently coloring at home. A perfect example is when the final color of the hair comes out orange, green, red or a mixture of all three, and that was *not* what you were expecting.

Colors Galore!

Most of the haircolors you will probably use will fall within the *warmness* of haircolors. These will contain the colors of red, yellow or blonds, red/orange and gold, which are mixed within the overall formula. The *coolness* of a color will contain blue, green and violet. Black is the only color you will use in this category because its base is violet. These colors, both warm and cool, are called *base colors*. One or more of them can be found in *all* permanent and semi-permanent haircolor. They are hidden in the formula and listed on every container of haircolor. You can stay within the parameters of all the rules, laws, and boundaries of chemicals as they apply to black hair, and still there will be hundreds of possibilities for you to try that are safe for your hair. Colors Galore means that there is no end to the list of things you can come up with. Any color you desire is possible, and you can have all the fun you want with them, but you must never break the rules as they pertain to haircolor or the chemical relaxer.

Q-Cards for Q-Tips

For accurate recording keeping, purchase a pack of 3x5 index cards and a file box to keep them in. Make notes on everything you use on your hair. Do this for every member of your family. Make a card with the names of the shampoos, conditioners, chemicals, haircolors and other products you use. Include information about each product, how to use it, the amount of time the product was left on the hair, the amount of product used, and so on. Be precise. The more information you put on each card, the better. Always refer to these cards and never do any work on your hair without having the necessary cards in front of you. This is the best way to get it right every time.

A Color Tip: To keep things simple, when choosing haircolor, select whatever shade and level you desire, and one that has a base color of red, yellow, orange and red/violet, which will add warmth or a wine flavor to the mix. Try to stay in the brown family of colors or medium and dark blond. If you decide to color your hair a lighter shade, levels 8, 9 or 10 which are light blond, very light blond, and lightest blond, always keep a blue or blue/violet base in the mix. This will stop the hair from having a "brassy" finish in the final look, which will complement your complexion, regardless to your skin tone. These are the better shades for beautiful black women, and the array of colors and possibilities of mixtures and formulas are endless.

When semi-permanent red and red/ violet color, which only coats the hair shaft, is added to those natural brown colors, the result will be some of the most beautiful tones such as Burgundy, Mahogany, and many lovely shades of reddish brown that are perfect for brown and yellow skin tones.

104

Red base color in brown tones, medium and light brown will always create beautiful warm browns. When red is added to any shade of brown, it will cause it to become warmer. If you choose a brown tone that doesn't have a red base,

- ❑ Purchase a bottle of red haircolor,
- ❑ Add ¼ ounce to the formula to achieve a lovely, soft, warm brown,

Keep in mind that *red haircolor*, and *haircolor with a red base*, are two entirely different things. The base color is never the primary color.

Permanent red haircolors are in a family of their very own. However, the base color can also be red, but it is *hidden* in the formula and will not be as noticeable as when you add ¼ once to the formula. The natural haircolor of most black women is at Level 1-black, Level 2- dark brown or Level 3- light brown, black being the most prevalent.

Level 1-black, as it applies to the hair of people of color, *does not* mean that your hair is black, even if you measure it and find the natural color of your hair to be close to that of Level 1. Your actual haircolor, although very dark, will be *darkest brown*. Knowing this will come in handy later in this chapter.

Blondes Have More Fun

This may seem like a contradiction to what I have said earlier, but if you wear your hair short, 1-3 inches in length, with or without chemicals, and you want to go blond, go for it. I have said many times in this book that you should stay away from bleach all together, and I have *not* changed my mind. If your hair is an inch short, you have nothing to lose. The same can be said if your hair is 2 or 3 inches, you have nothing to lose. Just condition well and often.

When chemically relaxing the *new growth*, be sure the product stays on the new growth as much as possible. Do not smooth the hair, simply apply the product and let it sit on the hair until the hair relaxes on its own. There isn't anything more beautiful than a black woman with blond hair—the look is truly sexy. It doesn't matter how dark-skinned, bright or light-skinned she is, blond hair on a black woman is simply beautiful. Use a conditioning lightener or bleach, and look for one that can be used on the scalp. Remember they work best when your natural haircolor is Level 4 or 5. Most bleach will only lift 4 or 5 levels. Add this to your natural level to determine the final result.

When Using Two Chemicals Always Consult a Professional

At times this may be necessary. If properly applied, the double chemical process can be a beautiful styling concept, however, certain precautions must be taken. If you want to change your natural haircolor to a darker shade, it will be very easy to do at home. If you desire to change your natural haircolor to any shade lighter, however, you will need help. This is because the formula must be applied ½ inch from the scalp for the first 20 minutes. Attempting this on your own could result in a mess in the end. Shamboosie suggests that when you need a retouch or a virgin application to go lighter more than 1 or 2 levels above your natural level, have the work done professionally. There are certain hidden color issues that only a master colorist would be aware of and should be able to address. Attempting this work yourself may cause a lot of problems and cost a lot of money to correct.

The Level System

Every color company's color systems and formulas are designed according to the Level System, which ranges from Level 1 to Level 10. Your natural haircolor may not *exactly* match one of the shades on the chart, but it will come very close.

Level 1 - Black
Level 2 - Dark Brown
Level 3 - Medium Brown
Level 4 - Light Brown
Level 5 - Lightest Brown
Level 6 - Dark Blonde
Level 7 - Medium Blonde
Level 8 - Light Blonde
Level 9 - Very Light Blonde
Level 10 - Lightest Blonde

A Color Tip: If you have already tried to do your own color and have made a mess of things, whatever you do don't try to fix it yourself, see a professional.

The Level System Chart was designed to determine your natural haircolor. It can also be used to determine how light or dark you would like your hair to be. Next to every level are several shades of the same color, many of which are warm and cool. The chart will say which colors are warm or cool and can be found at most of the major hair care product store locations. If you currently color your hair, to determine your natural color, compare the swatches to your *new growth*, which is the hair closest to the scalp.

Developers

You must have a good understanding of how developers work. The volume of developer and the amount of time you allow it to stay on the hair, determines the degree of damage it will do to the hair, especially when **ammonia** is also a part of the formula. The idea is to use the right developer for the job, apply the product, keeping an eye on it by checking it every 5 minute starting 10 minutes after the application. Then get it out of the hair as quick as possible.

Developers are sold in 4 different strengths 10, 20, 30 and 40-volume, in a liquid and crème form. One of the major mistakes made by professionals and non-professionals alike is thinking that *all* developers are the same. They think that "peroxide is peroxide" and that it doesn't matter which one is used. The truth is that it matters a lot!

The Way Developers Work

- ❏ Use 10-volume developer if you want to lighten the shade or tone of your hair 1 level, or if you simply want to cover gray and stay at your natural haircolor.

- ❏ Use 20-volume for two levels lighter.

❑ Anything more than 20-volume developer should never be necessary.

❑ From this point on all the work must be done by a professional.

❑ To lift three or four levels lighter will require 30 or 40-volume developers respectively. These higher volumes work best with blond haircolors from Level 7 to Level 10, and if you want to go lighter.

A Color Tip: Never use 40-volume developer on chemically-relaxed hair. The possible damage to your hair can be extreme and impossible to repair.

❑ When working with bleach or blond permanent haircolor, double the amount of 30 or 40-volume developer to each ounce of color or bleach to gain more lift and a faster lift.

❑ Developer can be purchased in creams or liquids. Liquid should be used to do a bottle application with a liquid lightener and permanent haircolor.

❑ The thicker cream developers should be used for a bowl and applicator brush application and with a powder lightener or bleach.

❑ Your measurements should always be exact.

If you want to color and lighten the shade of your hair only 1 level, when your natural color is Level 1-black, follow this procedure:

▼ Mix 2 oz. of 10-volume developer with 2 oz. of a color and shade of your choice.

▼ The color you choose should be 1 or 2 levels lighter than your natural haircolor.

▼ A 10-volume developer will be gentler and will still result in a subtle change.

▼ Because your hair is naturally very dark, changing it to a shade 2, 3 or 4 levels lighter, normally would require a 20 or 30-volume developer, which is more harsh on hair that has been chemically relaxed.

▼ It is best to use a lighter shade of color rather than a higher volume of developer.

▼ The timing should start after the haircolor or bleach has been applied, not before.

▼ Do a strand test first, and time every stage of the process.

▼ To do a strand test select a small patch or section of hair and apply some of the same formula you will be using when you actually color your hair.

▼ Start a half-inch from the scalp and apply the formula to the section, all the way to the end.

▼ Set a timer for 30 minutes and check the hair every 5 minutes.

▼ You can use up to 45 minutes for this strand test. Whatever the final processing is for the strand test, the timing for the full head of hair should be the same or at least close.

▼ Check the hair after the first 15 minutes and every 5 minutes thereafter. All of the formula should be removed from the hair as soon as you attain the desired color.

▼ Make a note of the time because it is the same amount of time that will be required for the rest of your hair.

▼ The timing should start *after* the color has been applied, not before.

▼ It is normal that the hair where the haircolor is first applied will develop first, and faster than the rest of the hair. This being the case, wet a towel with cool water and remove as much of the product from that hair as possible. It will stop the action of the haircolor. This is also the reason you should keep a close eye on the work in progress.

It is never advisable to change the color of your hair more than 3 levels lighter than its natural shade. However, if you must, your natural color and level should start at Level 4, and it will require a 30-volume developer. When the natural haircolor is darker, the change will be slight and subtler, unless a 30-volume developer is used.

Every bottle and tube of permanent haircolor will list the color your natural haircolor should be to get the shade you have purchased for your hair. All shades of Level 10 will be different when it is applied to hair that is a natural Level 5 or lower because these shades are darker. Level 10 will normally lift 4 or 5 shades but only when the natural haircolor is level 5 or 6. When Level 10-blond haircolor is applied to hair the natural color of level 5 and below, the final result will be a medium to light brown, at best. This means you cannot go blond from levels 1 through 5 by applying a level 10 blonde haircolor, only bleach will do the job. When the same shade is applied to levels 6, 7, 8, 9 using 30-volume developer, getting to Level 10 or blond is more possible. Whatever color you choose, if it is lighter than your natural haircolor, keep the following in mind.

▼ Let's say the shade you have chosen to color your hair is level 9, very light blonde

▼ Determine what your natural haircolor is and whether it is Level 5 or darker.

▼ Read the instructions on the bottle of haircolor to find out how many levels of lift to expect.

▼ Subtract that number from the level of your natural haircolor.

▼ Whatever the answer is, add it to your natural level, and it will tell you about what color your hair will be in the final result.

The Chemical Retouch

The retouch of the chemical relaxer, and permanent haircolor and bleach must be restricted to the *new growth only*, every time that each process is necessary. *A professional should do all of the work.* Be aware that there will be irreversible changes in the texture of the hair. A high quality shampoo and conditioner is required every 4 or 5 days to care for your hair, after the coloring, bleaching, and the relaxer retouch.

Lifting Haircolor with Haircolor

The Rule—Permanent haircolor is *not* designed for lifting the natural color of your hair. When necessary, this is a job for bleach or a lightener. Hair color will lift your natural haircolor, but it also deposits color at the same time, and the amount of "lift" is many times uncertain. There is no way to know exactly what the result will be. Also, permanent haircolor is *not* designed for removing artificial or unwanted haircolor from your hair. This means you can't color your hair dark brown, find that you don't like it, and use a haircolor of a lighter shade to remove it. It simply will not work.

Forget About It!

Remember this, if you desire to change your natural haircolor of Level 1 to Level 10 using a Level 10 haircolor (Blondest Blonde), forget about it. It will not work, and if you are thinking you can do it in two steps (Double Processing) by applying the formula, and processing it a full 45 minutes, removing the color, and re-applying fresh product for another full 45 minutes with hopes of getting to level 10 (Blondest Blonde) forget about it. It will not work. You will be breaking another one of **The Rules** by over processing the hair and it will fall out. You only want to use permanent haircolor at full strength, for the full processing time of 45 minutes, once. To refresh the color, use a semi-permanent haircolor the same shade or during a retouch application, it is safe to pull the product through to the ends of the hair the last five minutes of the processing time.

Removing Unwanted Haircolor

Artificial, permanent or semi-permanent haircolor can and should be removed with a color remover, an "uncolor," a lightener, or a bleach. If the color is semi-permanent, use an uncolor designed for removal of semi-permanent haircolor, and use a permanent haircolor remover for permanent haircolor.

Danger Do Not Enter

This is the best way to begin telling you about the use of bleach, which is now referred to as "lightener." This product should *not* be used in most cases, but it can be used on special hair types, textures, and hair lengths, if the hair is in good to very good condition. If a chemical relaxer is involved, stay away from bleach all together. Bleach and chemical relaxer hate each other, and a chemical relaxer will eat up hair treated with bleach in about five minutes. You could be completely bald before you get the relaxer out of the hair. So if you must go blonde, buy a wig. It is much safer.

Essential Hair Loss Equations

- ❑ The Curl + Bleach = Hair Loss
- ❑ The Curl + Permanent Hair Color = Hair Loss
- ❑ Relaxer + Permanent Hair Color the same day = Hair Loss
- ❑ Your Hair + Bleach = Hair Loss
- ❑ Relaxer + Bleach = Hair Loss
- ❑ No Shampoo + No Conditioners in the hair ever = Hair Loss

Bleach eats away at everything that is left in the hair after it has been permed or relaxed. It swells the hair shaft, it leaves it with a cotton-like texture, and it always over-processes the hair. If your hair is a natural Level 1or 2, and you want to be blond, the hair will have to be bleached twice, and this is not a good idea.

People often tell me I look like Isaac Hayes, because we are both bald. (I must admit he has a lot more money than I have, but I think I'm better looking.) If you ever use bleach in your hair and don't do it the wrong way, and if you leave it in the hair too long or mix it improperly, people will be telling you that you look like Shamboosie and Issac Hayes. There are too many of you looking that way already. Thank God for weaves.

This cotton-like change in the texture of your hair will be irreversible. In fact, at this point you can start to grow your hair from scratch. Your ability to stop the breakage will be practically impossible, no matter what conditioning treatment you use. My advice to you is that you stay away from bleach altogether. If you *DO NOT* use a relaxer in your hair, you may be able to get away with the use of bleach. But your hair must be in excellent condition, however, and it should be done professionally, with good products and conditioned very well.

Only The Strong Survive

The texture of your hair must be strong enough to support a perm or a relaxer and a **peroxide/ammonia** base permanent haircolor. The hair must be in top condition if you intend to bleach your hair, but you don't want to do that if you are wearing a chemical relaxer. All of these products will have a softening effect on the hair shaft, which means it will become even more porous or softer. This can be disastrous for some hair textures, but there are a few textures that can handle it with ease. Finding such textures is very rare these days because so many women of color are losing so much of their own hair.

Factors to Consider Before Lightening Your Hair

- ❏ The overall condition of the hair
- ❏ The strength of the peroxide
- ❏ The length of time the color stays in the hair
- ❏ The level of color change expected
- ❏ The type of product to use

- ❏ The training and level of expertise of the person performing the service

- ❏ Most important, how well you take care of your hair before and after coloring

- ❏ How often you shampoo, condition, and treat your hair

- ❏ What you use to shampoo and condition your hair

The Solution

You will need a thorough knowledge of the different types of haircolor and conditioners that are available if you intend to color your hair at home. It will be necessary to learn the proper way to use haircolor for the best results. Learn all of the rules, the do's and the don't's.

The Basics

There are basically two methods of applying permanent haircolor— a retouch and a virgin method.

Retouch Method When Doing the Work at Home

You will need a willing friend to do the color application. *DO NOT TRY THIS YOURSELF!* If you want to do the work at home, here is the correct way.

- ❏ Always apply permanent haircolor to dry hair.

- ❏ Separate and clip the hair up into 4 sections, parting the hair down the center, and from ear to ear.

- ❏ Starting in the back of the head with the first quarter section, outline the section with haircolor, to the new growth only.

- ❏ Make ¼ inch horizontal partings, and again apply the formula only to the new growth.

- ❏ Process until you have the desired shade or the allotted time.

- ❏ Rinse, shampoo, condition, and style as usual.

To refresh the mid-shaft and ends of the hair, the color can be combed through the last 5 minutes of the process, but you must accurately time the entire process. *Timing is the key.*

Heat exits your body mostly through your scalp, and body heat plays an important role during the process of a virgin application. If the natural color of the hair is to be lightened, and heat is added to the mix, it speeds up the action of the haircolor. One of the biggest mistakes people make, including many hairstylists, is to apply the color from the scalp through to the ends of the hair.

 A Color Tip: Let me warn you, this is not something you want to try, unless someone else is doing the work and you are the subject. A virgin method means the hair has never been permanently colored before.

Hot Roots

When changing your natural haircolor, going lighter, the body heat at the scalp causes the first half-inch of the hair closest to the scalp to lighten much faster and lighter than the rest of the hair. This is called *"hot roots,"* and the result is that the hair will have two shades. This happens because the formula should not be applied all the way to the scalp in this case. The hair in the scalp area will look like it's "on fire." Correcting this can be quite tricky, and will require the know how of an expert colorist.

The Virgin Method—This Is How We Do It

Here is the correct way. If you are going to lighten the hair, get a helper and remember to always apply permanent haircolor to dry hair.

- ❑ Separate and clip the hair up into 4 sections. Starting in the back of the head, make ¼ horizontal partings.

- ❑ Apply plenty of color, starting ½ inch from the scalp, all the way to the ends of the hair.

❑ After you have applied haircolor to all sections, set a timer for 20 minutes.

❑ Apply color to the ½ inch at the scalp.

❑ When color is applied to all sections, set a timer and process *up to* 45 minutes, this will include the first 20 minutes.

 A Color Tip: The term *up to* means, use as much time as you need, which is not always 45 minutes, but never more than 45 minutes. Use your own judgment.

Virgin Method with a Darker Color

Apply the haircolor from the scalp to 1 inch from the ends of the hair. The ends have been on the head longer. There may be split ends, the ends are more porous, they will absorb more of the color and come up darker than the rest of the hair. So always apply color to the ends the last five minutes of processing. If you are using a temporary, semi-permanent, or a long lasting semi-permanent haircolor, use this same method of application. Process the full allotted time, and rinse until the water runs clear, but do not shampoo your hair. Then condition and style as usual.

The Color Wheel

When the makers of haircolor begin to formulate their colors they decide first on the actual shades and colors. The colors are chemically structured and added to other chemicals, conditioners and essential properties. In order to do this the chemist must take into consideration what is known in the business as the "Color Wheel." The wheel begins with:

❑ Primary Colors, every color in the universe is derived from these 3 colors

▼ Blue, Yellow, and Red

❑ Secondary Color is a mixture of the primary colors

▼ Yellow + Red = Orange
▼ Red + Blue = Violet
▼ Yellow + Blue = Green

❑ Tertiary Colors are a mixture of the primary colors and the secondary colors

▼ Yellow + Orange = Yellow/Orange
▼ Red + Orange = Red/Orange
▼ Red + Violet = Red/Violet
▼ Blue + Violet = Blue/Violet
▼ Blue + Green = Blue/Green
▼ Yellow + Green = Yellow/Green

❑ Complementary Colors complement each other by canceling each other.

▼ Violet + Yellow = Neutral
▼ Red + Green = Neutral
▼ Blue + Orange = Neutral

Contributing Pigments (CP)

This is the one secret that has created more problems for the inexperienced colorist than any other. I would go so far as to say that most people are not even aware that contributing pigments exist in hair. These are natural colors that are *hidden* in the hair, they are called the *contributing pigment*. They are underlying colors that are exposed and *can only be seen during a lightening or bleaching process*. The contributing pigment cannot be seen during a coloring process if you are changing your natural color 2 or 3 shades because artificial color is being deposited at the same time the natural haircolor is being lifted or removed. However, the contributing pigment will always affect the final outcome of a coloring process also.

As the bleach begins to remove the natural haircolor, a shade of the contributing pigment is revealed at each level from Level 1 to Level 10. They are always the same. If your natural haircolor is Level-1 black, and the hair is bleached to Level-10 lightest blonde, the contributing pigment is exposed and is different at every level of change

117

between one and ten. Once the bleaching begins the colors of the hair will never return to the natural shades, they are gone forever. Also all of the contributing colors are the same regardless as to where your natural haircolor began on the scale. It is very important to remember this, if the hair is bleached past the level of ten, which is pale yellow. It is possible that all of the natural pigmentation has been removed, which is called blowout. When this happens it will be next to impossible to tone that hair. The hair simply will not accept any colors, permanent or otherwise.

Level 1 – Black / CP dark red brown
Level 2 - Dark Brown / CP/red brown
Level 3 - Medium Brown / CP/red
Level 4 - Light Brown / CP/red orange
Level 5 - Lightest Brown / CP/orange
Level 6 - Dark Blonde / CP/orange gold
Level 7 - Medium Blonde / CP/gold
Level 8 - Light Blonde / CP/yellow gold
Level 9 - Very Light Blonde / CP/yellow
Level 10 - Lightest Blonde / CP/pale yellow

A Perfect Fix

There is a color called neutral. Its base color is also neutral. Both the color and base are clear and not a color at all. They are neutral, and when a half-ounce of neutral is added to the overall formula, they will draw a balance between the warmness and coolness of the final result. This eliminates every thought you may have concerning contributing pigment and the possibility of an unwanted color in the final result. For instance, if you are looking for a beautiful warm brown, the neutral will block any cool tones that may be hidden in the formula and the hair, and vise versa. So what you will get is the color and shade you were hoping for. If the color you are using is at Level 6, the neutral color must also be Level 6. It works because the neutral color isn't this or that, it is neutral, and it works like magic.

How to Neutralize Unwanted Colors

Often when coloring hair, unwanted colors surface because some-one did not follow the rules. When this happens, you will have one of two choices. If you are lucky it will be a lovely color one can flaunt or you may simply neutralize the color altogether. Listed below are other colors that will neutralize each other.

❑ Red - Green

❑ Yellow – Violet

❑ Orange – Blue

❑ Red Orange – Blue Green

❑ Yellow Orange – Blue Violet

❑ Yellow Green – Red Violet

Now What Does All of This Really Mean?

Now that you know which colors neutralize one another, let's say you have colored your hair, and it turned out to be redder than you wanted. To get rid of the red or tone it down, purchase another color similar to the shade you used, but with a base color of green. The base color is always listed on the bottle, just below the name of the actual color and shade. As you remember, we learned previously that green neutralizes red, and vice versa. Follow this same principle when dealing with every other unwanted color.

Another way to deal with unwanted colors is to formulate the color to be applied so that it will neutralize the unwanted color during the process. These are called secondary colors.

❑ Yellow + Red = Orange

❑ Red +Blue = Violet

❑ Blue + Yellow = Green

If the hair turns out green or greenish, apply red for just 5 minutes. If it turns out yellow or gold, apply red mixed with blue to make violet, which will neutralize the gold or yellow tones. Use the same principles to deal with every other unwanted color. This system will work whether the haircolor is permanent, semi-permanent, or temporary.

The Tale of Scary Red

A client, who we will call Sonia, came in with bright red hair and said she couldn't stand to look at it another day. I lightly shampooed her hair. I then mixed blue and yellow, which made the most beautiful green haircolor I have ever seen. I showed it to Sonia and said, "This will do the trick." Well, I thought she would pass out from the thought of possibly having "green" hair!

It took me some time to talk her into trusting me to put this green haircolor on her hair. Finally, after much coaxing, she allowed me to apply the green haircolor to her hair.

I let it sit for a few minutes. As I checked to see if it was working, I made these awful facial grimaces, which caused Sonia much concern. (Of course, I knew this client very well, and knew that she was good-hearted and could take a joke.)

After about 5 minutes I rinsed, shampooed, and conditioned her hair. I was careful not to allow her to see the final result. (This drove her crazy, and I loved every minute of it.) Finally, she looked in the mirror, and with a sigh of relief what she saw was a beautiful warm brown! (We laughed about this on her many subsequent visits to the salon.)

Explore The Many Colorful Possibilities

The one ingredient in black, as it relates to haircolor, that restricts your ability to do what you want with your hair is the chemical relaxer. It is not an issue with white hair and other textures where relaxing the hair is not necessary. So changing the color of your hair from 1 to 10 shades and colors lighter is much more possible and safer. The key here is find those things you can do safely and be as creative as possible.

The concepts of coloring the hair and being as creative as you can are found in the many choices you have with temporary and semi-permanent haircolors. The possibilities are endless. With semi-temporary haircolors, no chemicals will ever come into play. Semi-permanent colors condition as they color and tone the hair. They only deposit color without chemically altering the texture of the hair, which means they can be applied the same day of the relaxer retouch.

Some Possible Formulas

❑ To apply a Level 10 Lightest Blonde, permanent haircolor to Level 1 Darkest Brown hair, use 30-volume developer and set for 40 minutes. This will lighten the hair possibly 3 ½ levels. Any semi color that is applied to the hair is called toning.

❑ Remember, once you lift or lighten your natural haircolor, you create a canvas on which you can paint any 1, 2 or 3 of hundreds of shades, tones, and colors.

❑ At this point and with semi-permanent haircolors you can place any color anywhere you want it. So any section, patches, or strands of the hair can be any one or any combination of 100's of possible colors.

From green, to yellow, a host of reds, golden colors, and browns. Red & blonde, black & blond and if the hair is synthetic, you can color it and place it in any section of the head you choose.

❑ Let's say that your hair is a Level 4 or 5 and light enough to do some very beautiful things with it. Jazzing from Clairol has many sexy colors that can change the total look of your hair. The wonderful thing about Jazzing is the colors are intense. Their staining properties are concentrated, and with hair this light in color, whatever shade of Jazzing you put on it, mixed with the color of your hair will produce some beautiful special effects.

❑ Try these sizzling colors. Spiced Cognac, Fuchsia Plum or Cherry Red. Spot place the colors or leave them on for only 5 minutes to produce just a hint of the shade. Apply, wait just 5 minutes and rinse, condition and style.

❑ If you wear the natural look, dreads, braids or an Afro, because there is no chemical relaxer involved you can be bit a more creative. One of the most beautiful things I have ever seen on a black woman is blonde hair. You must condition the hair regularly and use just the right bleach or lightener for the job. Shamboosie recommends BW2000 from Clairol. Follow the directions precisely.

❑ Try this, if you were to apply semi-permanent red with about a half ounce of blue/black, the gray hair will come up lighter in color and give you a beautiful highlighting affect. The same can be done with any shade or color as long as it is lighter than your natural haircolor.

The Aluminum Foiling Method of Application

1. Use the same formula, Lightest Blonde with 2 ounces of 30-volume developer to lighten the hair, only this time we will use a foiling method. This is not something one can do alone.

2. Cut about 12 pieces of aluminum foil, 3 inches wide and 8 to 10 inches long. We will only be working with the front sections of the hair, but the same process can be done all over the head. Make a part down the center of the head toward the front, and comb the hair to the left and right of the parting.

3. Now vertically part and separate a section of the hair about 2 ½ inches wide from the center part, down and in front of the ear on both sides. Clip the rest of the hair back and away from the face.

4. Starting at the top of the section, make a very thin horizontal part, about 1/8 of an inch, the full width of the section. Holding the ends of the hair with one hand, use the rattail end of the comb with an up and down motion, weave out small pieces of the thin section and separate it from the rest of the hair.

5. While still holding what's left of the thin section, fold down about a ½ inch of a piece of the aluminum foil on one end, place the tail end of the comb in the fold and place the foil and comb under the section of hair at the scalp, lay in the hair and fold down on the head to secure the foil.

6. While still holding the hair and foil, use an applicator brush to apply the toning semi-permanent haircolor to the section on the foil, and be generous with the color.

7. If the hair is longer than the foil, fold it into the foil as you paint the section.

8. Then fold the foil in half horizontally toward the scalp. Using the rattail comb to crease the fold on the left and right sides, fold the foil on both sides and have them meet in the center. Then clip the foiled section up out of the way.

9. Make the next section about ¼ of an inch think, twist it and clip it to the foiled section. The idea is to put a section of the hair without color between the foils.

10. Now repeat steps 5, 6, 7, 8, and 9 until all of the hair on both sides of the face is completed.

11. Time each section from 5 to 30 minutes depending on how much color you want the hair to absorb.

12. Remember, the color you use to tone each section can be any color, and any intensity you desire, but use only semi-permanent haircolor.

13. Remember that semi-permanent haircolor will only deposit color, they stain the hair and it is always temporary.

14. Always shampoo once and condition the hair after every service.

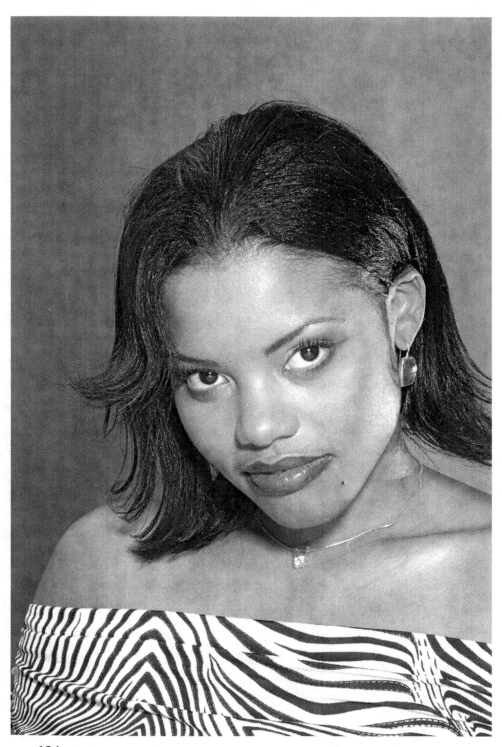

Chapter Eight

The System #1: The Sodium Hydroxide Conditioning Lye Relaxer

A Hairy Tale from Madam Erleen and Her Hairless Crystal Bald

Once upon a time a weird viper of hairy doom entered the house of many hairy fantasies to show his wares, while many of his victims were unaware of his devious deceptions.

This is a true story. A few years ago, I worked in a lovely upscale salon owned by a very well-known celebrity. One day the manager informed me a product representative would be coming to the salon to show a new product. The product was a relaxer that could be applied to hair that had previously been treated with permanent haircolor and a Curl. This would mean there would be three chemicals in the hair at once, (triple process). The claim was being made that this product could be used without causing any breakage. I knew very well that such a chemical would violate every law and the very theory of cosmetology. In other words, the creation of such a product is chemically impossible.

I urged the manager not to let this product be shown, and I thoroughly explained the problems such a product presented. I explained that there was no such chemical, and that if there were such a product, it would be very dangerous to use. Regardless to my strong objection, the management prevailed, and the representative showed his wares.

Approximately three weeks later, one of the stylists, Madam Erleen, decided to put what she had learned from the product representative to the test. A client came in with hair that was about five inches long all over, curly, and a lovely warm brown color. The client was excited about "coming out of the Curl," and in the end, that's exactly what she did!

Madam Erleen applied the chemical, and while doing the smoothing, it was noticed that the hair was beginning to shed. I train stylists that if shedding is noticeable, they should stop immediately, remove the chemical as quickly as possible, and neutralize the hair very well, then apply the best protein conditioner treatment. Unfortunately, Madam Erleen did not follow my directions.

So, as she proceeded, the client's hair began to come out by the handful. The chemical in this new product was actually melting the hair right off the head. Fear could be seen on the faces of everyone in the salon as they observed this disaster. Madam Erleen, however, continued the process, not knowing what to do next. She felt that she couldn't ask me what to do because the lines of communication between us had been closed. She had stopped listening to me weeks earlier.

As she began to rinse the client, she could see the client's hair being washed from her head right into the washbowl. In the end, the client was completely bald except for a few strands here and there. This was by far the saddest and most traumatic scene I had ever witnessed in all my years in the cosmetology field, and it made me feel sick inside.

Why am I Telling You This Story?

The good news is that you *can* find a hair care professional who will be concerned about the health of your hair, your satisfaction, and your well-being. It's up to you to seek out a hairstylist with that philosophy. It's your hair, therefore, you should want the best and the most qualified hair care service provider.

Remember to be very careful about what products you or your stylist uses in your hair. Don't believe everything you hear, and don't use every new product that hits the market. Utilize the advice contained in this book to answer your hair care questions and concerns. If you do so, you will save a lot of money, a lot of time, and a lot of hair! Learn about your hair and what's best for it, then your hair will live happily ever after.

Why the Real Lye is a Better Buy

Contrary to popular belief, a conditioning lye relaxer is the best relaxer for your hair and your scalp. It will leave the hair silkier and softer by conditioning as it relaxes the hair. The conditioning lye relaxer allows the hair to receive the moisture from conditioners it needs to retain its softness and to remain pliable. There is no calcium buildup and no extreme dryness, which you will always get with a no-lye relaxer. The conditioning lye relaxer leaves the cuticle layer of the hair healthier with every application (and that is no lie).

This means that when your hair is shampooed, conditioned and styled, it will have more body, bounce, and shine. These are terms seldom associated with black hair today. The use of the conditioning lye relaxer, will assist in helping your hair grow longer and faster, as long as you keep it well-conditioned.

The biggest problem with the no-lye relaxer is that the calcium buildup locks the hair, sealing the cuticle, and will not allow the hair to receive the moisture from shampoos and conditioners it needs to remain soft to the touch, pliable and capable of holding its curl and its style.

A Few of the Many Well-Kept Secrets

Product companies are always eager to introduce new products to the consumer. They are always aware of various problems women of color experience, so that they can create new products that address those specific problems. The created product will be so-named that the consumer can easily identify the problem it addresses, i.e. *dandruff* shampoo, *moisturizing* conditioner, **No-Lye Relaxer** etc.

Illustration: Most people "burn" every time they get their hair relaxed, and they believe that the reason is because of the lye content of the chemical. They will tell their hairdresser that they have a "very sensitive scalp." The truth of the matter is, everyone's scalp is sensitive to the relaxer.

To address this problem the product companies came up with a chemical that would take much longer to burn, if at all. They removed the lye from the relaxer, and replaced it with another chemical called *calcium hydroxide*. Then they printed the words **"NO LYE"** in large letters on the front of the packaging. They knew that the consumer would believe that no-lye relaxer is better for their hair, (which is a lie).

The intent was to get the consumer to buy, and consumers do buy these products to the tune of millions of dollars every year. Actually, the *real lye* is a better buy, because the no-lye relaxer is the most popular chemical relaxer on the market, despite its destructive capabilities.

Please Help Me Relax

I once worked in a salon where every client's hair appeared to be the same texture, very fine and fly away. If you think about it, it would be impossible for every client to have exactly the same texture hair. After a few weeks, I figured out what was happening. The owner had hired non-licensed persons to do the chemical services. She had taught them to comb the chemical through the hair every time when the new growth was all that really needed to be relaxed.

Many people believe they have to help the relaxer do its job, and this is where the bulk of the hair care problems begin. Each time the relaxer is combed through the hair, the hair is stretched to no return. This causes each of the hair strands to become smaller and smaller in diameter. When the hair is stretched, like an over-stretched rubber band, it becomes so thin, that eventual fall out is imminent. In order to perform a chemical relaxer service properly and safely, one must understand how the chemicals work.

Here is A Scary Fact

It is probably accurate to say that no two hairdressers apply relaxer the same way. This means that few of them were taught the proper way to apply the relaxer. When the relaxer burns the scalp and causes scalp sores, the problem is not with the lye that is in the relaxer. The problem is, and has always been, with the person applying the relaxer.

But The Tune That Follows!

Since most Hair Care Professionals do not understand how the neutralizer shampoo works, most of the time the client will end up walking out of the salon with a lovely hairdo, "**but the tune that follows.**" About 90% of the time the client leaves the salon with the chemical *still active* and *still working* in the hair. When the chemical is left to stop working on its own, it can take up to 24 hours after you leave the salon for it to stop working. That is enough time for the relaxer to eat clear through the hair.

The Ultimate Chemical Test

Once I tested the relaxer's effect on some strands of hair. I painted the hair strands with the chemical, wrapped the strands in foil, and left them overnight. The next day the hair strands and the relaxer were one. The relaxer had dissolved the hair completely. I realize this is scary, but when the relaxer service is performed correctly, there are seldom any problems.

There Should Never Be Scalp Burns

Believe me when I tell you that no one should ever receive scalp burns or scalp sores, and no one should ever experience extreme shedding. Scalp burns and shedding only happen because of a lack of knowledge on the part of the stylist. Add the reality of this to the fact that they also use the most dangerous chemical on the market to relax your hair,, and you can be absolutely sure of losing every strand of hair you have.

The Solutions Are Easy

Included in this chapter is a section called "**The System #1: Shamboosie's Proper Application Techniques**," which contains a step-by-step guide for properly applying the chemical relaxer. The System will cover everything in simple, easy-to-follow detail. If you learn the steps and follow them, you can do them at home with ease and with complete confidence.

When this step-by-step guide is followed exactly, there will never be any burns, no matter how many times the service is performed. This is your recipe for success, and it will work every time. No more scalp burns, ever.

Shamboosie Suggests:

- ❑ Always use a quality *conditioning lye relaxer*, no compromises.
- ❑ Purchase and use a timer.
- ❑ Most important, read The System #1 in its entirety before you begin.
- ❑ Make a copy of The System #1 and give it to your hair stylist. Insist that she use it when relaxing your hair.

You are probably wondering how you are ever going to convince your stylist to learn this innovative and safe method of applying the chemical relaxer. I promise you it will be much easier than you think…here's how.

This Is How You Do It

A *regular* client will visit the salon for a shampoo, conditioner, cut and style every 2, 3 or 4 weeks consistently. She will get a retouch and treatment every 6 to 8 weeks consistently. This means that as a *regular* client, you could spend approximately $1,000 to $1,400.00 a year on your hair, which does not include the purchase of Hair Care Products. Multiply this times 2 to 10 years. Hummm! It adds up, doesn't it?

Now figure out what you spend on your hair and your children's hair. Make a list of it and give it to your stylist. Then insist that she use The System #1 when relaxing your hair! I'm sure that once the stylist learns how this system really works, she or he will use this method exclusively. If you decide to have your hair relaxed at home, you will need the help of a friend. If you desire to relax your daughter's hair at home, the information in this chapter will teach you to do it the proper way.

The System #1—Truly A Mother's Helper
No Scalp Burns Ever—No Guesswork

The material presented in this and the following chapters are simple "how-to" procedures. They can be utilized by anyone who desires to learn the proper methods and techniques of chemical service applications, and the use of Marcel curling irons. My job is not only to tell you what to do, but also why it should be done, and what will happen as a result of doing it. It is also my purpose to give mothers the know-how needed to relax their daughter's hair at home, while at the same time, keeping their hair healthy, strong and growing.

In a family where there are many females, the cost of professional hair care services can be astronomical, possibly $200-$300 every six to eight weeks. Since so many of you are doing relaxers at home, it is important that you know the proper application method. My desire is to help you save as much hair and as much money as possible.

 A Chemical Tip: I recommend that unless you have help, you have this service and all chemical services done by a hair care professional, because when you do your own retouch, you can't see all of your own new growth well enough to apply the chemical only to the new growth.

When you do your own relaxer, you are forced to comb the chemical through the hair that has already been relaxed each time, just to get the new growth straight. It makes absolutely no sense to straighten hair that has already been straightened? Why straighten your hair over and over again until there is no hair left on your head? That is exactly what happens. If you must relax your hair at home, there is a way to do it correctly and safely, with no burns ever.

Requirements needed for chemical relaxer retouch at home:

- ❑ One chair with no arms and a soft cushy seat, which will be your resting place for about an hour.
- ❑ You will need one dozen small towels, two combs, rubber gloves, and a shampoo cape.
- ❑ You must have access to hot and cold running water.
- ❑ The right relaxer and neutralizing shampoo.
- ❑ A high quality conditioner.

The next requirement is number one in importance. Performing the service correctly and safely at home will require:

- ❑ Four human eyes, two looking down, and two looking straight ahead. The two looking straight ahead belong to the person on the receiving end, might that be you?
- ❑ You will also need four human arms with human hand attachments, two of them moving about and two just resting in your lap.
- ❑ The two eyes that are looking down will be able to see clearly all of your new growth, which is the only place the chemical should be applied.
- ❑ The two eyes that are looking straight ahead will find this task impossible to do.
- ❑ You will also need someone with the intelligence of a rocket scientist (big joke), who will be capable of reading, comprehending, and following the very simple, easy, basic step-by-step instructions outlined in this chapter.

Simply put, what you will need is the assistance of a willing friend. The friend will do the work, and you will just sit, and talk about all of the gossip you know, or watch TV, but do not read a book. It is important that you are the only one doing the talking. The helper should just listen and do the work. That's the price you will have to pay to look good. If you want to help out, reading the instructions out loud to your friend will be helpful.

 Shamboosie Says: The art of chemically relaxing overly curly hair involves knowing a few secrets about the way the chemical works, its effect on the hair, and what actually takes place throughout the process. All of the bonds in the hair, which cause it to be overly curly, will be altered or destroyed forever during the process.

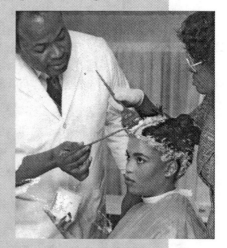

This is commonly known in the industry, however, what many are not aware of is that it takes between twelve to fifteen minutes for hair to totally relax, starting from the time the chemical first comes in contact with the hair. This will happen all by itself without the aid of a comb. It will happen even if the chemical is allowed to just sit on the hair for 15 minutes.

A tingling sensation will and should occur in the area of the first quarter section where the application began. At this point, you will have approximately two to five minutes to complete the service, and begin the rinsing process. Watch your timing.

Burn Baby Burn

Here are the ten most common causes of scalp burns:

1. Scratching the scalp with the fingernails a few days prior to having the hair relaxed. The itching that is often experienced is the scalp's way of telling you it's time for a retouch.

2. Shampooing the hair the day of, or the day before, the hair is to be relaxed. Make every effort *not* to touch the scalp or shampoo the hair a week before the relaxer service is to be performed.

3. Not basing the scalp. Most people, including professionals, believe that when the package says "no-base relaxer," it means you should not base the scalp before applying this very hot chemical, which is a lye relaxer. They don't seem to realize that this is basically the reason why the scalp is set on fire so quickly. *Always base the entire scalp before applying relaxer, and use a base that is designed for that purpose. See The Care Package.*

4. Leaving the chemical on the scalp too long. This is one of the primary reasons. If 100 people were to perform this service, it will be performed 100 different ways. The majority will leave the chemical on the scalp too long most of the time. (I can honestly say from personal experience, when the scalp starts to burn, it is not a good feeling, and I wouldn't wish it on anyone).

5. Having the service done just after sweating from exercising or swimming or doing anything to cause the scalp to become wet. Wetness of any kind will always cause the scalp to burn, even if you dry the hair. Wetness opens the pores of the scalp, softens the skin, and makes more sensitive.

6. Combing the chemical through the hair irritates the scalp and will cause the scalp to burn.

7. Using the wrong strength and the wrong type of relaxer for your hair.

8. The home relaxer kit, the "kitchen perm." The kitchen is defi-
    nitely not the best place to do this service because the facilities
    are not adequate, and there are safety hazards. However, if
    you must relax the hair at home, buy all of your products in
    separate containers, not in a kit. This way you can choose only
    the best. Read all of the directions on the package before you
    start, then apply The System #1.

9. This is the greatest reason of all. If the person performing the
    service does not know how to use the chemical relaxer, the
    application process will be guessing game.

10. You really do have a very sensitive scalp, most people do, but
    this is usually not the reason for scalp burns.

 A Chemical Tip: Timing is the key. Timing is the most
important phase of this process. Do not take this
lightly and be aware of your working time during the
entire application process. Buy and use a timer, please!

This Is How We Do It

Shamboosie's Proper Step-By-Step Chemical Application Techniques
Please read all of the instructions below, before starting.

❑ Section the hair into 4-quarter sections, down the center of the
head, and from ear to ear. Twist, and clip each section into place.

❑ When beginning the relaxer process, **DO NOT** apply relaxer
first around the face and hairline, and **DO NOT** apply the
chemical around all of the partings separating the quarter sections. To do this will indeed cause scalp burns in these areas
because the chemical starts to work the moment it touches the
hair and scalp. You want total control of this chemical. The
relaxer should be applied to each quarter section separately as
you go. Finish applying product to one quarter section before
starting the next. Start in the back of the head first, never
around the face first.

Chemical Tips:

1. When smoothing, do not maintain or smooth those partings between the quarter sections, only the horizontal parting of each quarter section. To do otherwise will cause the hair to separate down the middle of the head and from ear to ear in the finished look, and it could take a week or two to get rid of those separations.

2. Apply relaxer to the outline of the first quarter section in the back of the head. Start on the left or right side. This means the chemical should not be applied to any other areas of the head. Remember, each quarter section of the hair is handled separately.

3. Next start at the top of the first quarter section, and make 1/4-inch horizontal partings. Apply the relaxer to the upper side of each parting only, as you go along and use enough of the chemical to get the job done. This will add speed to the application process. The bottom side of the part will share the chemical on the top half of the parting when next part is made and chemical is applied to the upper side of that parting.

4. Handle each quarter section exactly the same way, with one exception. When applying relaxer to outline the two front quarter sections, it is very important to leave the area around the hairline and face for last. It should be applied to this area at the completion of each separate quarter section as you go. In other words, this area should be last, after all of the other hair has been covered at end of the third quarter section, and then at the end of the fourth quarter section.

5. The reason why chemical should not be applied first to the hairline around the face in the 3rd and 4th sections is because the hairline around the face is where the scalp and facial skin meet. Facial skin is softer, of a different type and is far more sensitive than the scalp, with many more sweat and oil glands. Facial skin will have a faster reaction to the chemical and burns will occur much quicker in these areas. Plus the hair around the face is always drier and more resistant as a result of daily washing of the face, and is usually baby hair, which is more fragile. This hair will be the first to go if, or when, breakage begins.

These rules do not apply when doing a Curl

Remember that the chemical relaxer starts to work the very moment it comes in contact with the hair, the scalp, and the skin. The idea is to properly straighten all of the hair without scalp burns and without over-processing or under-processing any portion of the hair.

The first application must be completed in ten minutes, about 2 ½ minutes per quarter section. Set a timer for ten minutes and work all of that time without talking. Your total concentration must be focused on the application and the time element.

Chemical Tips:

- ❑ When smoothing, **DO NOT COMB** the chemical through the hair, **DO NOT COMB** at all. Be gentle and work with speed, keeping the chemical in the area of the new growth only.

- ❑ Apply more cream as needed and cover every tiny piece of hair around the hairline and the back of the head (the nape area.)

- ❑ Again, using fresh partings start with the first quarter section working from the top.

- ❑ Make thin horizontal sub-sections, and apply additional relaxer where needed to the upper side of the horizontal partings only, for faster application.

- ❑ The smoothing is done as the relaxer is applied. Remember timing is the key.

- ❑ The third time through is smoothing only, about two minutes to completion.

- ❑ The person may feel a bit of tingling where the chemical was first applied, at this point. This is your signal that the hair is about ready to be rinsed and the possibility of scalp burns is eminent.

- ❑ Each application should be applied all the way *to* the scalp, but *not on* the scalp.

A Warning
Remember that the hair is very fragile while it is being chemically relaxed, and combing stretches the hair, which can't be seen with the naked eye, but will cause breakage. So don't ever comb relaxer through the hair. *The chemical will do all of its own work.* The second application will go much faster, it will take only about five minutes to complete.

You must use enough of the relaxer creme to get the job done, so don't be stingy. Smoothing is not done to straighten the hair or to help the straightening process. It is only used to help you determine if the hair is completely relaxed.

When the hair is properly relaxed, it will lay down on the scalp. If the hair is not properly relaxed, it will rise up slightly off the scalp as you smooth. When the hair is relaxed, it will feel silky and very soft to the touch. If it feels hard to the touch when it's time to remove the chemical, give it one or two more minutes. If the hair is not relaxed by the end of that two minutes, start the rinsing process anyway. If the hair is not properly relaxed, it will revert to curly or wavy after the first shampoo and conditioner a week later.

Remember, during a new growth retouch application, the hair to be relaxed is only the new growth, which is the hair closest to the scalp. The rest of the hair is already straight.

In basic cosmetology training, the students are taught to apply the chemical a ¼ inch off the scalp. This is not the proper way because the hair you want to relax is that ¼ inch of new growth. Doing so will cause under-processing. that ¼ inch of hair needs the full 13 to 15 minutes of processing time to be relaxed properly.

A Chemical Tip: Warning! When you are relaxing hair that has previously been relaxed with *No-Lye Relaxer* and the hair was not properly straightened, the no-lye relaxer will "lock in" the remaining curl pattern in the hair. When this happens, nothing, not relaxer, Thio, or anything else will be able to break this hair down and remove the curl. The only hair that will become straight is the new growth, the hair closest to the scalp.

Things to Remember

- ❏ Always examine the scalp for scratches and abrasions.

- ❏ Section the hair into four sections. The sections that are not being worked on should be clipped up and out of the way.

- ❏ Always base the scalp. Apply protective base to the entire scalp and one full inch around the hairline, ears and nape area, leaving no dry spots. Check it before you start.

- ❏ Use a base designed specifically for this purpose. Petroleum jelly or hair grease should never be used as they are too heavy and may interfere with the process. I recommend Vitamin A, D&E Scalp Oil by Dudley Products.

- ❏ Wear protective gloves at all times.

The Corrective Retouch and Virgin Relaxer

Applying a conditioning lye relaxer over a No-Lye Relaxer, (which I recommend) is called a corrective retouch. You can expect minimal shedding, but don't be alarmed. Do a treatment following the retouch.

For the corrective relaxer and the *virgin relaxer*, apply the chemical to the entire length of hair shaft, but remember timing is still the key. When it is a corrective relaxer, you begin and complete the process the same as any retouch. After smoothing the third time, apply the chemical by hand to the rest of the hair and smooth with your hands for only 3 to 5 minutes. Then begin the rinsing process.

The object here is to simply condition the hair that was previously relaxed with the no-lye relaxer.

With a *virgin relaxer,* use the same process as with a retouch except the chemical is applied to the entire length of the hair, one quarter section at a time. The smoothing is done with the hands until the hair is totally relaxed.

In every case, completing the service should take 18 to 20 minutes when using a mild, 22 minutes with regular, and 22 to 24 minutes when using a super relaxer.

Timing is Everything

The timing begins with the start of the first application, which is the very moment the chemical comes in contact with the hair, and the time ends with the beginning of the first rinse.

Relaxing Color-Treated Hair

Be sure to use a **mild** relaxer every time, no exceptions. The idea is to protect the color-treated hair, even if the new growth is not completely relaxed as straight as you would like it to be at the end of the process. Be sure to coat the color-treated hair with a styling gel or crème conditioner, to protect that hair before applying the relaxer and be sure you keep the chemical in the area of the new growth. All of this is an absolute must!

 A Chemical Tip: A Warning – Even if you were using a **super** or a **regular** relaxer prior to applying permanent haircolor to your hair, use only a *mild* relaxer from this point on or until you grow completely out of the haircolor.

The Rinsing Process—Set a Timer

The rinsing process should begin 7 to 9 minutes from the end of this 12 to 15 minute time period. After a total of 22 to 24 minutes, you must begin to remove the chemical starting where the chemical was first applied. So you will have to work with speed. This is the reason the helper should not talk during the process. Talking will slow her down.

The possibility of burning will occur between 20 to 24 minutes for most people, no matter how well you base the scalp. This is from the time the chemical first comes in contact with the hair, and should happen in the area where the chemical was first applied.

When most of the hair has been sufficiently straightened, the rinse should be initiated in the same order as the application of the chemical.

Starting with the first quarter section, rinse only this section thoroughly for 2 full minutes before moving on to rinse the next quarter section. Then rinse the second quarter section for two full minutes. (Set a timer for ten minutes and keep an eye on the clock)

After the second section is completed, rinse both sections again, for one full minute, before moving on to the third quarter section. This is a of total of 5 full minutes.

Rinse the third section for two full minutes. Then rinse all three sections for one full minute, the total time is now 8 minutes. Then proceed to the fourth section, and rinse this section with all the rest of the hair for 2 full minutes.

This is Why We Do It

Rinsing in this manner will allow sections two, three, and four to have sufficient time to completely relax before the chemical is removed or rinsed. All of the chemical was not applied to the hair at the same time, so the hair will not be completely relaxed at the same time, which means all of the hair should not be rinsed at the same time. It is also the only way to ensure that *all* of the hair will be completely and properly relaxed.

Chemical Tips

Towel blot all excess water after each rinse, and change the towel around the neck before neutralizing the hair. This will prevent breakage in the nape area due to residual chemical left in the soiled towel.

Proper neutralization and conditioning are essential for any finished look. This process is the most important part of this technique. It must be done the proper way every time, no exceptions and no compromises.

You must stop the action of the chemical. Failure to do so will leave the chemical to continue working for hours after the hair has been styled and finished. In that case, loss of hair is inevitable. You must towel blot all excess water from the hair after each rinse, so that the neutralizer shampoo will not be diluted.

When applying the neutralizer shampoo, use a generous amount. The lather should have the consistency of whipped cream. Do three shampoo applications, massage very well, and pay special attention to the nape area. Towel blot the excess water after each rinse, and leave the last neutralizing shampoo in the hair for five full minutes. Set a timer.

Apply the conditioner and leave it in the hair for a full 15 minutes. If the hair was previously relaxed with no-lye relaxer, and no haircolor is involved, condition the hair with Humectress Moisturizing Conditioner. If a dryer is needed, cover the head with a plastic cap and place under a warm dryer for 10 to 15 minutes.

Important Points to Remember

- ❏ During the application, never comb the hair in an effort to aid the straightening process.
- ❏ When smoothing always use minimal pressure or a very light touch, and try not to move the chemical around any more than necessary.

❑ Remember, it is the breaking down of the bonds that will relax and straighten the hair. It is a chemical process not a physical one. Let the chemical do the work.

❑ If breakage is noticed while smoothing, remove all of the chemical immediately and as quickly as possible. Treat the hair with a quality concentrated protein conditioner followed by a quality moisturizing conditioner designed for damaged hair.

❑ Remember, the person receiving the relaxer service should never be left unattended with the chemical still in the hair, at any time during this chemical process.

❑ If any discomfort is noticed, remove the chemical, even if the hair is not completely straightened. A sting, tingling, or an itch here or there is not the same as "burning."

❑ If there is a reaction to the chemical in just a small spot somewhere on the head, say a sting, tingling or an itch, use a towel to remove the chemical from that spot only, and spray some hairspray on the spot. The hairspray will cool the area. It will also give you about 2 minutes, maybe the time you need to finish the work. Continue to smooth and check the hair.

❑ If the hair is not in healthy condition, do a series of conditioning treatments 3 or 4 times for about 2 weeks, to make the hair stronger and to bring the hair back to a more healthy state.

Hot Stuff, Very Hot Stuff
If you should shampoo your hair and suddenly realize you were intending to have your hair relaxed. **DO NOT** dry the hair and attempt to apply the relaxer. Severe burning of the scalp is certain to occur in the first 5 to 10 minutes. Your scalp will be on fire before the chemical can be removed. The intensity of the burning will increase rapidly. The same will occur if you get caught in the rain, go swimming or do a shampoo the same day or the night before the retouch relaxer.

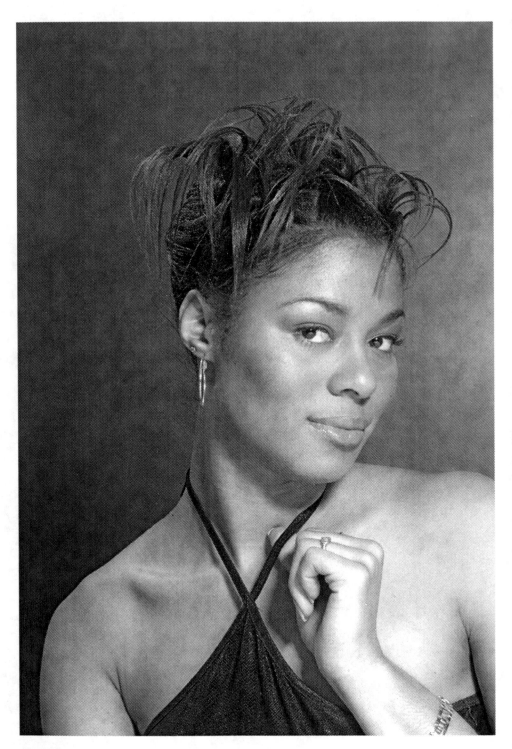

Chapter Nine

The System #2

Using Marcel Irons, Pressing and Curling with a Gentle Touch

- ❏ You will need a good haircut.
- ❏ Always apply setting lotion before drying the hair.
- ❏ Purchase a hair dryer with a comb attachment. When drying the hair keep the dryer moving.
- ❏ Never make the sections more than ¼-inch thick and 2 inches wide.

Hot Curling

I recommend using Dudley's Crème Press hairdressing and Dudley's Total Control (spritz). I have found them to work the best for the hot iron set. Curling with these products will insure that the curls will hold and last three to four days without having to roll, set, or re-curl the hair. Whenever re-curling is necessary, simply repeat the process, and use a small portion of Crème Press daily.

 Shamboosie Suggests: Allow enough time to do the work properly, and slow the process down. You do not have to dry your hair in the first 10 minutes, so take your time. Keep your eye on what you are doing. Start by spraying in pre-mixed setting lotion, and then dry the hair in small sections.

Blow-Drying the Hair

The reasons hair is often "puffed up" after drying is because most of the time you are in a hurry to get the hair dry. Also there is a chance that most of the hair "air dries" on its own. It is important to take the time to do it the right way.

You may need to spray a little more setting lotion occasionally to keep the hair damp, but not wet. The hair will dry straighter and smoother because you are drying from damp to dry. Any unwanted wave or curl in the hair will be very difficult to get out after you have allowed the hair to dry on its own. So keep the hair damp.

- ❑ Clip or pin-up the hair that is not being dried, to keep it out away from the flow of the heat.

- ❑ If a section of hair air-dries before you are able blow it dry, spray in a little water or setting lotion on the hair as you go.

- ❑ It is best to use a small plastic spray bottle about two inches tall that sprays a light mist. It will allow you to dampen the hair rather than wet it. Remember, drying the hair from damp to dry is the key to getting it straight.

- ❑ Use the comb attachment, put a little tension on the hair as you dry it and direct the heat only toward the hair that is being dried.

Getting the Hair in the Nape Area to Lie Down

When the hair is very short in the back, getting it to lie down is sometimes a task.

 Shamboosie Suggests: Keep the very short hair freshly relaxed, about every 3 to 4 weeks, but only in those very short areas. The hair will grow, and in as little as 2 weeks there will be new growth. The new growth is different in texture. It has some curl which tends to push the short hair out. The new hair simply will not stay down.

Setting for Bedtime

Shamboosie Suggests: Apply a little setting gel for short hair in the nape area. Comb to smooth the hair and remove any excess gel, using the index finger and a rattail comb. Tie the hair down with a folded scarf 3-4 inches wide. The scarf should be well secured, but comfortable, not too tight. If necessary, put a few rollers in the top or hot curl the top in the morning.

 Shamboosie Suggests: When using little rollers with the sponges and clip attachments, wrap the sponges with plastic wrap to protect the hair because the sponge rollers are known to eat away at the hair and cause the hair to shed and break.

Styling with Rollers

The best rollers to use are cylinder-shaped rollers for wet setting or when using a setting gel. They come in 6 or 7 sizes and 2 different lengths. You can purchase a set of rollers containing various sizes.

When the hair is wet, it will cling to the roller and allow a smooth set. If necessary, use end papers to help control the uneven ends. Begin the set in the front, and leave the bang section without roller for styling later. Make sure the hair around the face is evenly set, and use the appropriate size roller according to the length of the hair. If the hair is short, set as much as you can on the rollers, smooth the rest with gel, tie this area down with two neck strips and pin in place. Dry the hair, preferably under a hood dryer. You will also need the proper clips to hold the rollers and the set in place.

Where is the Base of the Hair?

The base of the hair is where the hair and scalp meet, like the base of a lamp. The base of the hair controls and dictates everything the hair *will* do, *can* do and everything you *want* the *hair to do*. The hair strands of a section of hair a ¼-inch thick and 2 inches wide will create a base strong enough to make a section of hair 3-4 inches long stand straight up, lean to the left or to the right, lean slightly forward or slightly backward.

This Is How We Do It

Add a smidgen of Crème Press to all of the strands of hair in the section. Then spray hair with Total Control styling spray. Place a hot curling iron at the base, close the iron, and hold it for three seconds, then remove the iron. This will lock the base of the hair in a stand-up position or in any of the other positions by "directing" the hair. Move the iron to the ends of the hair, and curl the ends.

Understanding how the base of the hair works will enable you to position the hair for styling during the drying process. I usually accomplish this with my brushes, curling irons, and blow-dryer with a comb attachment. For example, if you want the hair on the right side to move back away from the face, over the ear, and to lie close to the scalp, dry the hair so that it will fall that way.

In your mind's eye you must visualize everything you want the hair to do, one section, and one curl at a time. If you can *see* it, you can *achieve* it. Hairstyling is just that simple. The hair is dried "on base" when it exits the scalp and immediately lies down on the scalp.

❑ Separate the hair in as many sections as you need to give you control of the hair. Twist and pin up each section. Dry each section, making the hair do what you want it to do. Simply push the hair in the direction you want it to go.

❑ If you want volume and movement on the right side, place the comb in the hair at the base, and pull straight out away from the scalp.

❑ If you want the hair to move toward the face on the left side and the bang section to fall on the face, continue to dry the hair, moving it in a circle around the head. This will throw the hair back off the face on the right side, and forward on the face on the left side and forehead.

❑ When curling the hair that lays on the face and forehead, simply "bump" or slightly bend the ends with a large iron.

❑ If you want the hair to stand up, or if you want to add some height, place the comb at the end of the dryer in the hair at the scalp, and pull straight up. This should be done while the hair is still damp.

❑ If you want all of the hair to move off the face, simply dry it that way.

❑ All that is left is to put in the curls, and create the style, one curl at a time.

❑ Always apply setting lotion before drying the hair, and apply hairdressing and spritz after the hair is dried.

❑ Practice to perfect these techniques, and you will be able to create any style.

Most Important

❑ It is very important to place each curl at the end of the hair only. "C" curls will do. However, if you desire a curlier look, put in full circles. When the hair is 8 to 10 inches, shoulder length or longer, begin curling the hair closest to the face and stack the curls with the sections 2 inches wide and ¼-inch thick.

❑ When the hair is dry, apply Crème Press in dime size portions to all of the hair, which should take about 3 minutes.

❑ Remember to be light-handed when applying oils.

❑ Spray Total Control styling spray in all of the hair, and comb through with a large tooth comb, and let it dry.

Remember, hair loses its natural ability to hold curl when it is chemically relaxed. Hot curling is used most often for styling hair that has been chemically relaxed. You will be able to create curls that will hold for days on end, if you learn to use the proper techniques, the proper tools, and the proper styling aids.

Pressing The Issue

The hot pressing method of straightening the hair is one of the oldest methods of straightening overly curly hair. It's amazing that the art of pressing the hair is still around, but it is regaining some appeal. Today it is being used as an alternative to chemical relaxers. Women who don't want their hair relaxed, but prefer not to wear it in natural hairstyles, are opting for the "press and curl."

Hot Combs

Hot combs are made in two sizes and two shapes. I prefer the small iron for doing most of the work; these are the ones with slightly curved thin teeth. They allow you to get as close to the scalp as possible without burning. The small comb is for work in tight areas and for working with hair that is very short. The larger comb is for longer, thicker hair, but a professional can use either of the two and do the job well.

This Is How We Do It

❑ This is another process that requires two people, which means you should not press your own hair because possibility of scalp burns increases when you "do it yourself," unless you have done it for years and know how.

❑ The hair can be pressed in small, individual sections or, if you are good at it, you may start anywhere on the head, as long as all of the hair has been pressed when it's all said and done.

❑ Remove any distractions. Pressing hair is an "eyes on" technique that requires concentration. You do not want to talk to anyone or watch TV while pressing hair.

❑ The iron is very hot, so please be very careful, and take your time.

❑ The comb should be hot, but not hot enough to burn out the hair.

❑ Hold the ends of hair with your free hand, and place the teeth of the hot comb into the hair about 1/4-inch off the scalp.

❑ Keep the comb in place, and rotate the back of the comb down, as close to the scalp as possible, without touching the scalp. The pressing or straightening of the hair is done with the back of the hot comb. The teeth of the hot comb simply separate the strands of the hair. This should be done with one continuous motion.

❑ Pull the comb through the hair once or twice to "soft press the hair," and two to four times, to "hard press" the hair. The Crème Press will leave the hair smooth and silky but not oily.

❑ After all of the hair has been hot pressed, you can either roller set the hair or hot curl to style. If you decide to hot curl the hair, spray the hair lightly with the styling spritz, and curl as usual.

The hair should be pressed every 1-2 weeks to maintain. If there is permanent haircolor, a curl, or chemical relaxer in the hair, *do not* hot press the hair. Not even to press the new growth because this will cause the hair to break and fall out. The heat from the hot iron will burn through the hair and cause breakage at the *line of demarcation*. Pressing is for virgin hair only.

Proper heating of the irons is the key to getting the desired "finished look." This could be very difficult to do at home. Heating the Marcel irons on top of your kitchen stove is very different than using a stove made for this purpose. On the kitchen stove the irons will always get too hot, and the heat will be uneven and more intense. This could burn the hair right off the head.

How to Take Complete Control Over the Heat

- ❑ Fold a cloth hand towel three times and wet it with cold water. Be sure to leave some of the liquid in the towel. It should be very wet, but not dripping. Place this towel near the stove for easy access.

- ❑ The first time the iron is placed in the stove it will take about 2 minutes to heat to a temperature hot enough to curl hair.

- ❑ The way to test the heat is to lay the barrel of the curling iron on the towel soaked with cold water before putting the iron into the hair. This way you can make sure the iron is not too hot and is ready for curling.

- ❑ The key to controlling the heat is in the sound of the iron touching the towel soaked with cold water.

- ❑ If you will listen carefully, the sound you will hear when a curling iron is too hot for curling, is a "blistering" sound, loud, like dropping cold water into a hot pan.

- ❑ If the sound you hear is more moderate and less blistering, it means the iron is safe to begin curling the hair. The iron will only be hot enough for curling about three curls, and then reheating will be required. It should only take 20-30 seconds to reheat, but be sure to test the iron *every* time. The 20-30 seconds should be just enough time to section the hair, comb the section, and add a smidgen of Crème Press and spritz. Comb through the section, and curl that section of hair. It will happen automatically with practice.

Important: Marcel irons are for *professional use*. I do not suggest using them at home unless you know how to use them properly.

Cooling the Curling Irons

❏ If you continue rubbing the iron on the wet towel, it will quiet the sound, cooling the iron in the process. If the sound goes away completely, the iron will become too cool to curl the hair, and must be re-heated and cooled again. Getting the iron to the right temperature for curling will require some practice. What you always want to hear is a slight "hissing sound," which will mean the iron is safe to curl with. Occasionally, you may need to replenish the cold water in the towel.

❏ *Never leave the irons in a hot stove unattended.* The irons will become too hot to handle. If you were to touch them, you won't be touching anything else for about 3 months. If the irons are accidentally left in the stove too long, do not touch them with your bare hands. Use a thick, folded, *wet* towel to remove the irons.

❏ Never put over-heated irons in cold water to cool the iron. This will cause *warping,* and the irons will be useless.

❏ Put the irons in a safe place to cool. Be sure they are out of the reach of children and away from anything that could catch fire.

No Smoking Allowed

If you see smoke coming from the iron while you are curling, it means you are burning the hair, which will result in breakage. The iron should be as hot as necessary; however, smoke should be almost invisible. Every stove that is made for the purpose of hot curling and pressing will heat differently, some faster and hotter than others. The cost of these stoves is between $35 and $50. Curling irons and pressing combs will cost between $15 and $35, depending on the type of iron, name brand, and place of purchase. Choose the stove and irons you are most comfortable with.

Do Not Touch to Test

Never touch the stove or the irons to determine if they are hot enough for curling hair. Do not touch the stove even if you know it is unplugged or cold. There are two ways to turn off the stove and the curling irons—turn the switch to the *off* position, and unplug both the stove and the curling irons.

Curling at Home

The safest way to curl at home is to use an electric curling iron. There are some very good ones on the market. I do not suggest using a curling iron with a knob for adjusting the heat, because this type of iron gets too hot and you could end up with one or two pocket curls, the kind you burn off the head. You may need two curling irons, one with a barrel the size of a dime, and another the size of a quarter. If your hair is shoulder length or longer, you may want to purchase one with a barrel that is 1-1/2 inch in diameter. I recommend professional electric curling irons because they will do a better job, heat better, and they will last the longer.

Styling with The System#2 requires practice and patience, but if you take your time, in a short period of time, curling will become easier.

There are many different kinds of curls. Even the slightest bend in the hair is considered a curl. The more times the hair is wrapped around the barrel of the iron, the curlier the look will be in the comb out. The key to styling with the Marcel irons is in being able to put the exact kind of curl, the exact shape or bend, in the hair and place each curl in the exact position for the desired style.

Be Gentle, Like Holding a Baby

Always grip the iron gently when curling, like holding a baby. It is not necessary to apply pressure or to squeeze the irons. Remember to flap the iron slightly and constantly. The heat and roundness of the iron will do all the work. Curling this way will allow the iron to move smoothly, and easily through the hair, and will allow the hair to slide easily through the barrel and flap of the iron. Remember to grip the curling iron gently, like holding a baby. The heat and roundness of the iron will make the curl, there's really no need to squeeze.

154

The Types of Curls are Endless

Some examples of types of curls are:

- ❑ Standup curls, with or without a stem
- ❑ Curling on-base and off-base
- ❑ C-curls
- ❑ Full circles
- ❑ Multiple circles
- ❑ Figure 8's
- ❑ Long and short soft waves
- ❑ Shirley Temple or Spiral curls

There are also waves made with a flat iron. The flat iron is very popular and it will create a slight bend in the hair. There are about 20 different sizes of Marcel irons, and each type of curl will change with the size and type of iron used.

Important: Flap and Turn the Iron

- ❑ Whenever you are curling, flapping of the iron should be slight and constant, with just enough space between the barrel and the flap to allow the hair to move through the iron.
- ❑ You may pause for a second to allow the heat and the roundness of the iron to form each circle.
- ❑ There should be just enough of an opening between the barrel and flap to free the hair to move through.
- ❑ At the same time the iron is being turned in place, if done properly, the ends of the hair should end up inside of the curl, free of the barrel and the flap.
- ❑ This will allow the iron to be easily removed from the hair without disturbing the curl. Remember, practice makes perfect.

Stand-up Curls

If you desire to create fullness and body on top,

- ❑ Pick up each ¼ inch section of hair, and with the barrel facing toward the back of the head, close the iron on the base of the section close to the scalp.

- ❑ Then loosen your grip, and move the iron to the ends of the hair and make one circle.

- ❑ If you are right-handed, the curls should begin on the left side in the crown area. Make two rows of curls, the second row to the right of the first.

- ❑ Work from right to left until all of the hair in the top is curled, or make one row of curls followed by another.

- ❑ Start with an iron the size of a quarter, if the hair is 2-4 inches. Use a smaller iron as the hair gets shorter. Do not try curling hair ¼ inch or shorter. Gel and dry the hair close to the scalp.

This method will create a style off the face with the curls moving toward the back of the head. To move the style toward the face, simply reverse the curl pattern and curl the hair forward. The section of hair closest to the forehead and hairline will require little or no curl on the ends of the hair only.

Curling On and Off Base

Pick up the section and place the iron at the ends of the hair to curl "off base." For curling "on base," comb the section of hair straight up, and place the iron close to the scalp on the base of each section.

C-Curls

This type of curl is simply a half circle placed at the end of each section of the hair much like the turn at the end of a walking cane. This curl can be performed with any size iron, and is the curl used in the majority of hairstyles when the hair is cut in a short style. When the hair is cut in a shoulder-length bob or longer, use a large curling iron or a flat iron to bump the ends of the hair. If you want curl in any of the hair, put one or two circles in that hair. If a softer curl or

156

slight bend in the hair is what you want, put that in the hair. Simply place the amount of wave or curl in the hair you desire.

In every case, all of the curls should be in line and even with each other, from very short to hair that is 2 ½ to 4 inches in length. If the hair is thick, place two or three curls evenly on top of each other.

Try to imagine a string running through each of the curls like pearls in a necklace. Notice that no matter which way you turn the string of pearls; each pearl will follow one in line after the next. So it is with curling, the curls should flow and follow one after the other and in line with each other.

 Style Tips: After your hair has been given a cut of your choice, here are a few tips that will help you when styling your hair at home. Remember set aside enough time and then take your time and practice.

▼ Pick the hair up in ¼ inch sections, ½ inch wide.

▼ Coat each of the sections from the scalp to the end with a smidgen of Dudley's Cream Press.

▼ Spray on some Dudley's Total Control styling spritz.

▼ Place the very ends of the hair in the iron at the bottom of the barrel, as close to the handles of the iron as possible, not at the end of the iron.

▼ Roll two full circles of the hair evenly around the barrel and flap of the iron.

▼ The iron should remain closed.

▼ Keeping the hair in place, continue winding the hair diagonally around the barrel of the iron, until all of the section is around the iron.

▼ Rest for a count of three. Open the iron slightly, releasing the hair. Turn the iron once, and remove it from the hair without disturbing the curl. Repeat this process to completion.

C-Curls are used in most layer cuts for a fuller, smoother comb-out. For most layer styles, use an iron the size of a quarter for longer hair, and smaller as the hair gets shorter. Full circles are used for a curlier look. Change the size of the iron, as the hair gets shorter.

Multiple Circles and the Figure 8

These types of curls will only work when the hair is six inches or longer. Pick up very small, ¼ inch, sections one inch wide. Place the iron midway of the hair shaft. Holding the ends of the hair with the free hand, slightly flap and turn the curling iron, allowing the hair to move easily through the barrel and flap of the iron, while winding the hair into the curl around the barrel. Usually the hair will be curled from the ends to the scalp. This is the most difficult of curls to perform. It is very important not to simply wrap the hair around the barrel of the curling iron. The hair instead is *wound* into the curl, so that the hair moves through the barrel and the flap of the iron.

Long and Short Smooth Curls

These types of curls are perfect for longer hair. Place a large iron in every section, turn slightly, and simply slide the iron through each section of the hair. With this method of styling there is almost no curl in the hair. If more curl is desired, place the iron at the ends of the hair and in line with the cut. Then turn the iron once, hold for a count of 3, then turn the iron 180 degrees, allowing the hair to slide through the iron and remove the curling iron. Comb each curl with a small tooth all-purpose comb.

Shirley Temple Curls aka Spiral Curls

You must have long hair to wear these curls. This is an old curl pattern and style that was named after the legendary child star Shirley Temple Black. She was a singer and tap dancer more than 40 years ago. For many years, little girls wore Shirley Temple curls, usually on special occasions. Today these curls are referred to as Spiral Curls.

Smooth curls, long and short soft waves, and very slight bends in the hair are mostly made with a very large curling iron or a flat iron. For shoulder length hair or a bob, pick the hair up in ¼ inch sections and curl the very ends of the hair. Make the curl at whatever the angle the hair is cut.

 Shamboosie Suggests: Select a good spritz, but not one that creates a firm hold. Choose a styling cream or hairdressing that is not oily. Oil causes the hair to shine for about one hour before the set falls out. This is because oil expands with the heat from the scalp, and will soften the set, causing all of the curls to fall. By the way, never use grease on your hair. I recommend Crème Press hairdressing, and Total Control holding spritz both from Dudley's Products.

This is How We Do It

Hold your hand in front of you horizontally with the fingers together, side-by-side, and imagine each finger as curls stacked one on top of the other. This is the way the curls should look. They should be the size of the iron used, about 2 inches wide, and if, possible they should touch each other. It does not matter if you are curling horizontally, vertically, or diagonally, and it doesn't matter if you are left or right-handed.

If you are right-handed, always curl from left to right. This means when you make your first vertical row of curls, the next section of curls should start to the right of the previous section of curls. If you are left-handed, you should do the opposite. Follow the same method no matter where you begin the curling process. This is called "systematic curling," The System # 2.

Curling in this manner will allow you to line up all of your curls, regardless of the size or shape, which will make the comb-out easier with a perfect finished look. If the hair looks good when the curling is finished, it will also look good when it is combed into the finished style.

If the hair is to be styled away from the face, start the curling in the back of the head, and continue toward the front. When the style is toward and on the face, the curls nearest the face should be curled first. All that is left is to decide if the curls around the face are to be soft, laying on the face, bumped (slightly turned at the ends of the hair) rather than curled, full circles, or flat smooth curve. Be creative.

See The Finished Look Just Ahead

The art to styling is to see the finished look in your mind's eye, even before starting the shampoo. If possible, try to see all of the components required to obtain the finished style. Components such as the cut, direction of blow-drying, the positioning of the hair for the set, whether hot curled or roller set, should all be in your mind before you start. After shampooing and conditioning, and while the hair is still wet, spray on some setting lotion to soften the cuticle layer. This will make combing and removing the tangles easier before drying the hair.

The Key

The key to styling while curling is to build the style systematically, one curl and one section at a time. Place the exact curl in the exact position for the style. If you follow this method, the comb-out, regardless to the style you hope to accomplish, will be as simple as ABC.

You've Got Me Curling in Circles

If you cut a lemon or an orange in half, you will see lines leading to the center. When cutting a cake or a pie, most people will start the cut in the center and cut to the edge. When two cuts are made, what you have is a slice. Part a circle of hair in the crown of the head four inches wide, and find the center of that circle. Next, part or separate the hair with a rattail comb from the parameter to the center of the circle. Make a second parting ¼ inch from the first part to the center, and what you will have is a section of the hair in the shape of a triangle. Pick up the section, comb it, and curl the ends.

Continue to do the same thing until all of the hair in the circle is curled. This is the system to use in curling all of the hair on the head in a circle, when making a turn around the ear, or when the curls are vertical on the side of the head and you wish to end up curling horizontally down the back of the head. You can use this method anytime you need to turn slightly or otherwise.

Making the Curls Hold and Last

When the hair is relaxed, it loses its ability to naturally hold a curl.

First, the styling Crème Press is applied lightly to all of the hair, in dime-size portions with the palm of the hands. Use a very light touch, apply sparingly, and be sure every strand is covered. Use as much of the crème as you need, but only in dime-size portions.

Next, spray all of the hair generously with the Total Control spritz, and comb through the hair with a large tooth comb. Dry the hair completely, and apply extra Crème Press where needed while curling. In most cases, the curls will be soft to the touch but will hold for 2 to 3 days, maybe longer. (I have had many clients whose curls would last a week and longer without rolling or re-curling the hair.)

Remember to position each curl, and allow the finished curled set to cool completely before combing out. Do not comb after each curl. Always use a very large tooth comb that has 3 or 4 large teeth for the comb out, and comb the hair in as few strokes as possible.

This will allow several strands of the hair to hold together, supporting one another, and the curls will last longer. Using a fine tooth comb will cause too much separation of the hair strands, and the curls in the set will fall out.

Important: Be gentle with your grip on the hair. This will allow the heated curling iron to do all the work. If sticking occurs, loosen the hair from the iron with the tail of the rattail comb, and continue curling.

The curling irons are designed so that the roundness of the irons and the heat will get the job done. No pressure is ever needed, so be gentle. The rest is art.

Pressing the Issue—The Right Way to Hot Press the Hair

Much has been written about black people wearing their hair natural and chemical-free. Some say that it is an expression of African pride and heritage.

Pressing and curling or wearing the hair natural may be chemical-free options for some people. However, relaxers, curls and other chemicals will continue to have a wide appeal. Let's face it, the natural look does not appeal to every woman.

In the old days, when pressing her daughters' hair, sometimes mom would put too much oil on the hair. Then the hot iron would melt the grease, causing it to also become hot. The grease would pop onto the scalp and cause real pain.

What made the whole ordeal even more threatening was that whenever mom would get a little too close with that iron, although she was being very careful, she would accidentally burn the scalp, forehead, the ears or and neck. Each time she would say how sorry she was and then tell you to sit still and stop squirming so much. You could hardly wait until the whole thing was over. Pressing and curling the hair should never be such a painful experience.

Using Spritz

A spritz is not a hairspray, but it will hold the set or the curls when used the right way. However, when used alone, spritz can leave the hair very hard and dry to the touch, which is not good for women of color. Spritz contains alcohol, and this dries the hair out.

Hard Pressing and Soft Pressing

Hard pressing will last about a week, and the soft pressing will last 2-3 days.

Pressing the Hair—This is How We Do It

1. Shampoo and condition the hair with quality products.

2. Towel dry the hair to remove as much water as possible.

3. Spray on some setting lotion to soften the hair. The setting lotion will soften the hair and close the cuticle layer, making the hair easier to comb.

4. Detangle the hair using a large tooth comb. Separate hair into as many small sections as possible.

5. Pin each small section up and out of the way. This will make blow-drying the hair much easier. Begin combing the first section toward the scalp, starting with the ends of the hair. Use a very large tooth comb to remove all of the tangles.

6. Next, using a blow-dryer with a comb attachment, dry each section as straight as possible.

Water with Nowhere to Go

Important: Water in the hair will air dry quickly because there is nowhere else for the water to go. The hair cannot absorb the excess water. The problem with this is that whatever natural curl or wave pattern is in the hair will surface when the hair dries, and this curl will be impossible to remove without moisture. You want to make sure the section of hair you are working with has some moisture in it before you begin drying it. You want to keep moisture in the hair to be able to dry it from wet to dry. This is the only way to get the hair straight.

Drying the hair from wet to dry will help to remove as much of the wave from the hair as possible, which will not be possible if the hair is allowed to air-dry. Begin drying around the face, and completely dry each small section before moving on to the next. The key to doing it well is in taking your time. Set aside enough time to do it the right way.

Slow the process down. When your arms get tired (and they will), take a break, watch a little TV, have something to drink. Then spray a little water and start again. You can do this as many times as needed.

When all of the hair is dry, use Crème Press from Dudley's, in dime-size portions. Apply to all of the hair, from scalp to end, and be sure the cream is on all of the hair. Then section the hair into as many small sections as possible to press and straighten the hair.

It's Time to Get Serious so Let's Press On

❑ Starting around the face, pick up each ¼ inch section of hair.

❑ Take your time and be very careful. This is a very hot iron, and to do a good job, this hot comb will have to be placed very close to the scalp.

❑ Place the hot comb in the hair as close to the scalp as possible. With a little pressure, press and pull the hot comb through to the ends of the hair. You may need to do this a couple of times to get the hair silky smooth and straight from the scalp to the ends.

❑ Move to the next section and repeat the same process until all of the hair has been pressed and straightened. When using any hot iron or hot comb, it is very important to do all of the work with the tip of the irons. This will give you more control of the iron and of the hair.

Black is Truly Beautiful

Every product will change the texture of the hair somewhat. Therefore, it is important to know precisely the best conditioners, shampoos, relaxers, permanent haircolor and other products that are necessary to care for and protect your hair after those changes.

Proper hair care is a topic of grave concern to many, and there is an urgent need to dispel all myths and misinformation about hair that seem to prevail. Women want real solutions to real problems, and they want them NOW.

Beautiful Black Hair: Real Solutions to Real Problems, addresses the hair care problems of the black woman in simple, easy to follow detail. Use it to assist you when caring for your hair and the hair of your family and friends. Make this book a gift to your friends and love ones.

If black is *truly* beautiful, and I believe that it is, I want to do everything I can to solve as many of your hair care problems as possible. I want to help make you more beautiful so that you can be the best that you can be. Remember, when you look good, you feel good, your self-esteem soars, and you're ready to face the world!

 Show and Tell—The Video

A video has been produced for Systems included in this book featuring an easy-to-follow explanation of each procedure followed by a demonstration of that procedure. The video called "Curling with Simplicity," covers everything found in this chapter including pressing, curling and hairstyling. It features fifteen different ways to do crimps, and the proper use of styling combs. The video also shows how to do comb-outs, and instructs on the proper tools to use, and the proper use of oils, sprays, lotions and gels. You will learn how to do it all with a gentle touch.

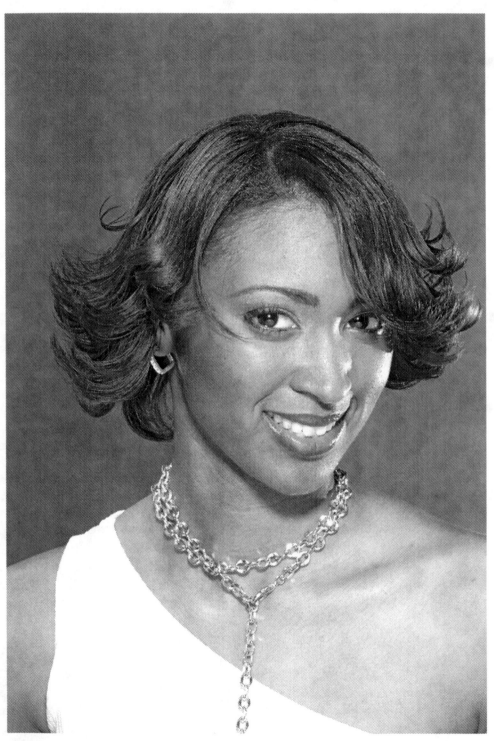

Chapter Ten

Getting It Together:
Rethinking the Hair Care Routine

Everything Must Change, Nothing Stays the Same

My Hair Just Won't Do Right!! Why?

There are several reasons why your hair can become difficult to manage at home.

1. This could be due to the lack of proper conditioning, over a long period of time and you could be experiencing shedding or breakage.

2. Perhaps the curls won't hold, or there could be too much oil in the hair.

3. If you have been using permanent haircolor at home, the hair could be over processed from misuse, which is true in most cases.

4. The hair may be weak.

5. You may have had a poor haircut, or a fresh relaxer retouch, which sometimes causes the hair to appear thinner, as if half of the hair was lost in the process.

6. You may be experiencing frizz, lack of body, bounce or fullness. Such words you seldom hear anymore because black hair is so dry and stiff from using No Lye Relaxer kits.

7. The hair may be puffed up.

8. The hair may be extremely dry, or there may be too much moisture in your hair.

9. You may have had a poor haircolor job, or you could be experiencing problems resulting from use of home relaxer kits or too many different chemicals in the hair at the same time.

10. Use of the wrong kinds of chemicals, putting in your own chemicals, and use of cheap Hair Care Products, will all create problems with your hair.

11. You may have had your hair serviced by an inexperienced stylist whose work was not up to par.

12. Perhaps your hair has been shampooed with regular facial soap instead of a pH balanced shampoo.

13. There may be a calcium build-up, or perhaps a medication you are taking has left a coating on the hair. If so, this will have an affect on your hair.

Any of these reasons can be the cause of badly damaged hair. The list could go on and on, but real solutions are available in this book.

Product Knowledge and Usage

The Pink Stuff

This is a two-in-one curl moisturizer and oil. Remember when using this product and others like it on dry sets, that when you are wearing the hair hot curled, blown dry and styled with a round brush or a roller set and styled, the oil shouldn't be used at all. The hair should never be oily. When the hair is oily, it will separate, and will not hold its curl. You could end up looking like you are having "a bad hair day."

Remember, oil and grease are not for the hair. There are very light oils designed especially for the scalp, which should be used lightly every three or four days.

In the past, The Pink Stuff was made primarily for use on the curls. Now it is being used to relieve dryness in the hair. The reason it doesn't work too well is because you are probably using too much and for the wrong reasons. It just makes the hair heavy and greasy-looking. If you must use this product, remember to use it only on the curl. I cannot stress this enough.

Because of the many chemicals and other Hair Care Products used on the hair, the cuticle layer of the hair undergoes some degree of change, causing the hair to appear dull-looking.

If you must add some sheen to the hair, it is best to use a cream hair-dressing that has high quality moisturizers, proteins, and very little real oil or grease in its formula. Any sheen or shine you are able to create will be very short-lived. With a creme hairdressing, the amount of oil in the formula is minimal. This way you can never use too much oil, and the hair will be nice and soft.

Setting Gel

There are many setting gels on the market, and as I have stated repeatedly, quality is the key. You may have to spend a little more money to get a gel that doesn't flake or dry the hair out. Keep in mind that setting gel is not glue, it is gel, and it works in the hair, not on the hair. It can be used every day, but should be shampooed from the hair at least once a week, followed by a very good conditioner.

Your setting gel should not dry the hair out or cause the hair to become hard to the touch, but it should leave the hair soft, even if the hair is set in a smooth mold. If the hair dries hard, find another gel. In molding the hair, the gel should be in all of the hair, but any excess should be removed. This will cut down on the possibility of flaking.

Hands Off Please!

Once the gel dries in the hair, spray on a little Total Control spritz and the set should hold all day. Clear gels are usually better because they can be applied to hair of any color. Once the hair is set, keep your hands off the hair during the day, but do check it from time to time as you would any hairstyle. Rubbing the hair constantly will cause the mold to separate and pieces of the set to rise up. So keep your hands off the hair. also apply a dime size portion of Crème Press.

This Is How We Do It: Using Setting Gel to do a Roller Set

❑ The best time to do this is an hour or two before you go out or to work. To set the hair, each time you pick up a section of hair to place on a roller, add just a smidgen of setting gel.

❑ Roll the hair and use a roller clip to hold the roller in place.

❑ In order to do this daily, you will have to get an early start in the morning.

❑ A good time to set the hair is after you have washed your face. Set the hair, and it will dry in the time it will take you to get dressed and put on your makeup. ("I'll say a little a little prayer for you.") Remember use just a smidgen.

❑ This type of set should dry in about an hour and comb out beautifully.

❑ Remember when setting the hair on rollers; don't pinch the ends of the hair together. Pinching the ends and allowing the hair to dry this way will cause separation in styling the finished look. The exception is if this is the look you want.

❑ Comb each ¼ inch section so that the hair is the same width from the scalp to the ends, about 2 inches wide. Setting gel can also be used for smoothing the nape area. Use a rat-tail comb and the index finger to comb and smooth the hair. Tie the hair down with a wide scarf, and the hair should set in about an hour or overnight. Other areas where gel can be used are the hairline, bangs and sideburns.

Hairspray

Hairsprays are finishing sprays. In the early days of my career, I thought hairsprays would really hold a finished set. However, after awhile, I realized that regular hairsprays are not for holding. It took me about ten years to find a holding formula that would really work and not leave the hair hard or dry.

I use hairsprays to tie up loose ends and flyaway strands of hair that will not cooperate with the style. When combined with a fine tooth comb, and a very light touch when combing, the hairspray can become one of your best styling tools. It can also be used to help the hair cling, add fullness when backcombing, and comb smoothly into place while sculpturing a pin up or up-do.

This Is How We Do It

Let's say you are doing a pin-up or an up-do. After the hair has been backcombed or teased, spray in some hairspray to help give you a very smooth finished look. Remember, be gentle when combing and comb only the surface of the hair, the outer most strands. This will insure that the finished set will be smooth and quite lovely.

Spritz

This product is not a hairspray, but will hold the set when used the right way. When used alone, spritz can leave the hair very hard to the touch, which is not good for women of color. Most spritz has alcohol in its formula and will dry the hair out. Today we have softer formulas that will allow you to use as much as you need. A creme hairdressing must be used to offset this dryness caused by alcohol. I recommend two products, Crème Press and Total Control Styling Spritz. They go together like a horse and carriage.

Oil Sheen

This product is simply grease in a spray can. A can of oil sheen should last you about twenty years. I know you think I'm joking, but I'm not. If used properly, a can of oil sheen really can last a very long time. Most hairstylists working in the salon will go through two to six cans per year. This is far too much oil. As I said earlier, *grease is for the scalp and not the hair.* Multiply six cans of oil sheen by ten stylists in the salon, and "grease is the word."

Your stylist sprays your hair with oil sheen in hopes that it will leave your hair pretty and shiny, and it does. The problem, however, is that the stylist wants to see the shine immediately after spraying. This is not a good idea because the stylist sprays a lot of oil on the hair. Sometimes the fog from the spray is so thick you can hardly breathe! The stylist has to find something to fan the fog so that you can catch your breath.

The hair will be shiny and greasy, but the set will fall out before the end of an hour, maybe even before you pay your bill, and leave the salon. Oil Sheen is a finishing sheen, and should be used very sparingly—one or two very small puffs over the hair, holding the can twelve to sixteen inches from the hair, allowing the mist to fall lightly on the finished set.

The shine (radiance) from the oil sheen should be seen moments later, after the light oil has settled and dissolves or melts into a light sheen on the hair. This normally takes about five or ten minutes. Oil sheen can also be used to base the scalp when the hair is kinky, short or very tightly curled, before applying a relaxer, or if the hair is to be texturized.

Oil Gloss

This product is an even heavier form of oil, which is used for hot curling with a styling spritz. Some are coated with a wax and dry to glassy gloss. I don't like to use them myself, but I believe them to be wonderful when used at hair shows, on stage, in competitions, and on "extraordinary" hairstyles which I call "showpieces."

Once You Start, You Must Never Stop

Once you chemically relax your hair, everything from this point must change. You can never stop relaxing your hair or it will break and fall out. If you should wake up one morning and say to yourself, "I am going to just stop using chemicals in my hair," or "I am never going to put another relaxer, permanent haircolor, or a curl in my hair." If any one or two of these products is already in your hair, the very day you decide to stop, be prepared to experience hair loss at an alarming rate. All of these chemical processes will change your hair in such a way that your hair actually becomes weaker over time. Most of your breakage will happen because the newly grown hair so much stronger, the two will separate and break at the point where the two meet.

Once you start to lose hair, stopping the process is very difficult. The loss of hair is inevitable, however, in a few cases, stopping the loss may be possible. The truth is that only the application of a relaxer will stand any chance of stopping the breakage.

Hair Today, Gone Tomorrow

So you say, what changes? With the relaxer the bonds are broken down. Many are destroyed forever, and there will no longer be a wave pattern or curl in the hair. In other words, the" kinky stuff" is gone forever. The hair will become porous and many times very dry. With permanent haircolor, the hair becomes very porous, softer, and weaker, but in a different way. This means the hair now has the ability to absorb more moisture than ever, and it will soak up anything that is applied to it. At this point, you now have two new changes happening in your hair, and the two have one thing in common. They both are causing softness in the hair.

Using a relaxer will require a change in the way and type of shampoo and conditioner you use. Add haircolor and it will all change again. If you do not properly care for the hair in any of these conditions, it will shorten the life of the hair and its ability to remain on your head.

This is exactly what has happened to the majority of you, and it has happened many times. This permanently changed texture cannot be reversed. A quality moisturizing high protein conditioner used regularly will be vital in caring for the hair.

On The Cutting Edge

Usually such an expression means *new, a fresh idea, unique* or *something that has never happened before*. Does this sound like some of the haircuts you've had over the years?

I once witnessed a client explaining to her stylist the way she wanted her hair cut. She said, "Cut my hair very short in the top and little longer on this side." "Cut it a little shorter in the back left side, and while you are cutting my top, don't leave me much of a bang section. Then make the right side a little longer than the other side and leave me a clean spot around temples and in the nape area." The stylist was puzzled, and asked, "Why do you want your hair cut that way?" The client said, "Because that's the way you cut it the last time I was here.!"

This is a typical scenario, but one I hope you have never experienced. The truth is finding a stylist who cuts well is not so easy, but it is possible. If you get a good haircut, you will have a much easier job of maintaining the style at home and keeping your hair looking great every day.

When I was a teacher of Advanced Cosmetology at the country's only university of cosmetology in North Carolina, one of the most difficult subjects I had to teach was Haircutting. My teacher in basic training told me the only way I would ever learn to cut hair would be to cut every chance I got.

She told me to cut everyone who sat in my chair, and if they didn't want their hair cut, I didn't have to do their hair. After more than 20 years, I have come to realize that to become a good cutter requires a bit more than that.

To cut well one must learn *all* of the basics and many of the advanced techniques of professional haircutting. This requires much training, much hard work, and much dedication. Often, some members of the cosmetology profession will not take the extra classes, or watch haircutting videos, and will not diligently practice the techniques until they are perfected. If they do learn the techniques they must then be used to cut every hairstyle as perfectly as possible, every time. The client is entitled to *nothing less*.

Who Will Make the Cut—It's Not Easy

Thank goodness there are many fine professional haircutters out there. Your job is to find one. The person who cuts your hair does not necessarily have to be the same as the person in the salon who styles your hair. Of course, finding one person who can do it all is ideal.

When you have achieved the look you want in a haircut, stay with that stylist and never let anyone else cut your hair. If your stylist is not available, don't take a chance with someone else cutting your hair because if that person doesn't do a good job, your stylist will not be happy with you. It could take one or two years to get your hair back to where it was.

Can They Cut the Cake?

The key to knowing whether or not your stylist is a great haircutter is in the stylist's ability to see the "finished look" in the mind's eye as early as the shampooing and conditioning stage. The stylist should be able to give you the exact haircut you desire. If your hair is easy to style and manage after the cut, at home, you will know that a professional cut your hair. Remember, a good haircut should be designed to accentuate all of your lovely features.

Cut a Little, Grow a Little More

It is my job to make the client's hair, damaged or otherwise, look as good as possible. Over a period of one to two years, the client and I must do all that is required to grow a healthier head of hair. This will require some work but the same work should be done in any and every case. If I were to cut off all of your damaged hair, what would be left to style? I can make damaged hair look really good with ease, while at the same time cutting a little and allowing a little more to grow.

Haircutting Tips

❑ Check out the very best salons in your area. This does not have to be a black hair salon. Remember to always do what is best for your hair. Simply walk in and ask for the best haircutter in the salon. She may not be the best stylist.

❑ Have the ends trimmed as often as necessary, every four to six weeks is best. If your hair is healthy, this will mean very little hair will need to be cut.

❑ Never allow the hair to be cut very short in the temple areas if you are thin in the areas around your hairline. Wear your bang sections and the hair around your face longer to cover the bald or thinning area around the face. Your stylist will know what I mean.

❑ Don't allow razor cuts, they look nice, but the ends will be cut on a slant, which will promote split ends over time.

❑ If you've been wearing the same hairstyle for a long period of time, you may want to consider a different look. This could do wonders for your appearance and give your spirits a boost, too.

❑ Don't ever try to cut your own hair. You will cut some areas too short, and once the hair is gone, it will be too late. This will make styling your hair at home extremely difficult. There are also some people you should include in the "don't let" category. Don't let your sister, momma, best friend, a neighbor, the mailman…you get the idea, only professionals, please!

❑ Ask for pictures of how the cut will look or possible cuts to choose from, and be sure to consider the shape of the face in the pictures and the shape of your face. They should be similar.

A Myth is a Lie in Disguise

Some Examples of Myths and Misinformation

- ❑ Wearing a curl will cause the hair to grow.
- ❑ Braiding the hair promotes hair growth.
- ❑ Running hot water on the hair and scalp will make your hair grow.
- ❑ There is lye in a No-Lye relaxer. The fact is, there is no lye in a No-Lye relaxer.
- ❑ Shampooing too often is bad for the hair.
- ❑ Sleeping on your back will cause the hair to shed in the nape area.
- ❑ Egg is a good conditioner for the hair. This one could really "stink."
- ❑ There is such a thing as a "kiddy curl" or a kiddy relaxer made specifically for kid's hair.
- ❑ A shampoo and conditioner-in-one is a healthy way to condition the hair.
- ❑ Oil and grease will relieve dryness in the hair.
- ❑ The no-lye relaxer is a better relaxer for your hair.
- ❑ Hair color will remove haircolor from the hair.
- ❑ You can stop using relaxer any time you want to.
- ❑ One can do a relaxer, curl, and haircolor safely at home and in the salon. This one might be possible with my help.
- ❑ The scalp burns from relaxer happen because the scalp is "sensitive". It should never happen.
- ❑ Putting blond haircolor on black hair will lighten the hair to blond.
- ❑ It is okay to use bleach on hair treated with relaxer.
- ❑ It is okay to switch from a curl to a relaxer.

❑ White stylists can't do black women's hair.

❑ Black stylists can't do white women's hair.

❑ Bald temples are hereditary.

❑ Black is the natural haircolor of most people of color.

❑ Mayonnaise is a good conditioner for your hair. It is true that mayonnaise contains properties that sound like they would work well for hair. However, with all the good Hair Care Products on the market, why use it? Go with the real thing. You need to know for sure the product will work, and nothing beats the real thing.

❑ Vinegar will remove chemicals from the hair. Once a customer came into the salon for a relaxer. She had been wearing a curl and had recently washed the curl out of her hair with vinegar. Nothing I said to her changed her mind and I can assure you, I did not put a relaxer in her hair. Don't believe the myths and don't take heed to misinformation. The opposite is usually the truth.

The Tool Box

I have been privileged to work in many salons over the years. My co-workers are always amazed by my collection of tools of the trade. I consider myself to be a comb collector, and I am constantly searching for unique and different combs to add to my collection. I have more than 300 combs of different sizes, shapes and colors.

I have hundreds of perm rods and rollers, and an assortment of brushes, sheers and other tools, all of which I need to get the job done. When I travel to do the large hair shows, I carry along what I have named the "Porto-Salon." This is actually a toolbox on wheels that contains everything I need to do my work. Many times my colleagues will ask to me to borrow my tools (and of course I refuse). I believe that every true professional should make it a priority to be equipped with all of the tools needed to do the work.

Tools of the Trade

Although it is unlikely that one would ever need 300 combs, some basic tools are necessary to do a good job of proper hair care. The use of professional tools will make the task a lot easier. A good beauty supply store will have all the tools you will need, and they will be able to answer your questions and offer suggestions. Here is a list of what you will need for home care and maintenance.

Combs:
- ▼ 6 Rattail combs
- ▼ 2 Large tooth combs with 8-10 teeth and a handle
- ▼ 1 styling comb with no handle and only 4 large teeth
- ▼ 2 Hard rubber large tooth combs
- ▼ 2 10" hair cutting combs

Brushes:
- ▼ 1 Cushion brush
- ▼ 1 Vent Brush
- ▼ 1 Round Brush

Irons:
- ▼ 2 or 3 Curling Irons with different barrel sizes (1 ½", 1", and dime size), electric or Marcel

Miscellaneous Tools:
- ▼ 1 dozen each Hair Pins, Bobby Pins and Roller Pins
- ▼ 1 box Duck Prong Clips
- ▼ 1 Plastic Applicator Bottle with a spout
- ▼ 1 Plastic Spray Dispenser Bottle (Press/Spray)
- ▼ 1 Full Set of Rollers (Cylinder Shaped)
- ▼ 1Box of Double Prong Roller Clips
- ▼ 1 box End Papers
- ▼ 1 Shampoo Cape and Styling Cape
- ▼ 1 dozen Towels (salon)
- ▼ 1 Pair of Cutting Sheers (spend about $40)
- ▼ 1 box Butterfly Clips
- ▼ 1 Small Duffel Bag (to store it all)
- ▼ 1 pack Paper Neck Strips
- ▼ 1 Hand Held Mirror

The Waiting Game

It's Saturday morning, and you have a full day planned, with errands to run, shopping, and all sorts of things to do. Unfortunately, your first stop is an 8 o'clock appointment at the beauty salon where, believe it or not, you have got to wait.

The salon opens at 8 AM, and you are on time, but you are wondering why there are so many people in the salon at this early hour. Well, your stylist intentionally "over booked" just in case someone didn't show up for their appointment. This morning, however, everyone showed up. Saturday is the busiest day, and the salon takes the last customer at 1 o'clock. You've been waiting almost two hours now, and all your stylist has done is had her assistant shampoo and condition your hair, and put you under a very hot dryer for 20 minutes. (Of course this was done only after you have been sitting there for quite a while glancing at your watch.) By this time you are really "steamed." This is done to make sure that you don't walk out until your hair is finished, even if you have to wait for 5 more hours.

Then you hear your dryer cut off (thank goodness that's over, it was very hot under there.) Wonderful, there you are, waiting for another thirty minutes before the assistant checks to see if you are "well done." This is the kind of thing that makes you want to look somewhere else to have your hair done, but you would just be starting the whole process all over again.

Seated next to you is another client who is just "cooking away" under a hot dryer, and she is talking so loud everyone in the salon can hear her every word. She is talking loud in order to hear herself because the dryer is making so much noise. She says, "I've been here for hours, and all I'm getting is a set." While you are still waiting, you look around the salon to see that everyone has the same expression on their faces. It's the look, which says, "If I ever get out of here, I am never coming back." Then you see it…a sign on the wall, which says, *"WE TAKE WALK-IN'S."* Can you believe it! No wonder you've been waiting for hours.

The truth is it should never take all day at the salon to have your hair shampooed, dried and curled. The solution here is simple,

Saturday is not the best day to get your hair done. Try to schedule an appointment earlier in the week.

With that in mind, if possible, schedule your appointments at off-peak hours. Plan to take off work early or take a long lunch break. Sometimes you can get an early appointment before work, or perhaps report in to work an hour late. You can also make your appointments after 5:00 p.m. on weekday evenings, to avoid " the Saturday waiting game."

Whenever you make your appointments, be sure to tell your stylist how much time you will have, and stress the importance of getting you out on time. When all else fails, that salon across town you've always wanted to check out, go ahead and check it out! It may be the best thing you have ever done.

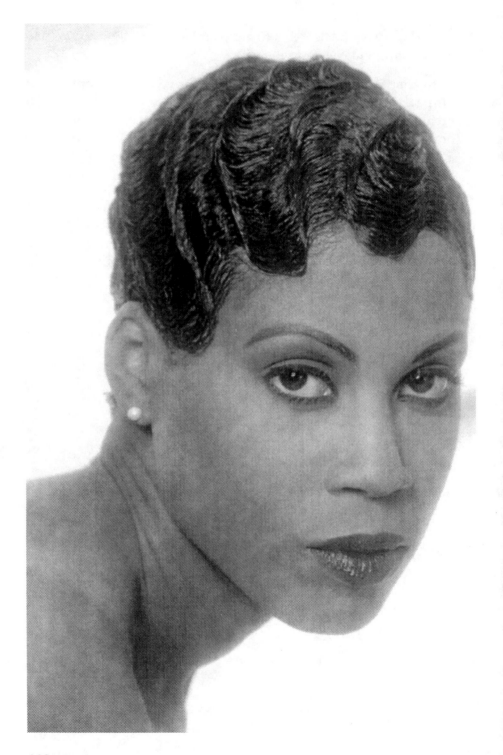

LOVE Your Hair

People will believe almost anything if it makes just a little bit of sense. There is a well-known quote from the Bible, "Money is the root of all evil." In that statement lies the reasons so many of us have a spiritual life that is in the same condition as our hair, but thank God this too will change with time. The actual quote includes the word, "love," "For the love of money is the root of all evil."

Some of you believed the first quote just as easily as you believe much of what people tell you about how to take care of and have that beautiful head of hair you used to have. The simple little four-letter word, **"LOVE"** will change everything for you, and the whole thing will make a lot more sense. For the love of your hair is the root to having a beautiful head of hair. **"LOVE"**

Thank you for allowing me to share with you this expression of my love. It comes with God's love and His blessings for you and your family.

Shamboosie

L Learn the basics.

They are easy to remember and they will never change. Learn the names of products, what they cost, when to use them, and what they will do for your hair. To know is a blessing.

O Observe the techniques.

Be aware of everything your stylist is doing to your hair. Open your eyes. Take note of the application methods that are being used. You need to know what is going into and coming out of your hair.

V Value healthy hair.

Appreciate, respect, treasure and admire the advantages of having lovely hair. Get as much of the right information as possible and put it to the test, it will work.

E Enjoy the results

of understanding the right things to do for your hair. Now that you have learned what it takes, you can have beautiful healthy hair every day. It's easy if you will simply **LOVE** your hair.

Special Acknowledgments:

Tony Rose, Publisher, Editorial Director
Samuel Peabody, Associate Publisher
Yvonne Rose, Senior Editor, Photo Stylist
Lisa Liddy, Cover and Interior Design
Shamboosie, Hair Stylist and Style Director
Deesha Prichett, Main Cover Model
Leslie Renee Milton, Cover Model Make-up Artist
James W. Laster, Cover Model and Style Gallery Photographer
Wayne Summerlin, Photographer (Conclusion)

Hype Hair Models: Deborah Williams, Derica Williams, Deesha Prichett, Tangela Bond, Michelle Green, Arvella Morton, Keisha Besay, Venus Buchanon, Asua M. Johnson, Katrina Lyles, Ashunta R. Sheriff, LaReece Darton, Leona Khap, Schelle Foster, Jeanita Valentine, Peggy L. Charles, Marsha Griffiths, and Bucarni Simms

Hype Hair Models, Make-up, and Hair Stylist Coordinator: Jackie Love

Hype Hair Stylists: Francis Silva, Leslie Milton, Lisa Prescott, and Sharon Alexander of Done Up! Salon

Make-up Artists: Ashunta Sheriff, Leslie Renee Milton, and Patricia Campbell-Stevenson

Chapter 1: Model, Egypt Lawson/Photographer, Dwight Carter

As always, Amber Books gratefully acknowledges those whose time, patience, help, and advice have contributed to the success of our literary efforts: Donna Beasley, founder, the Chicago Black History Month Book Fair and Conference; the IBBMEC; the nation's African-American bookstores; our wholesalers and distributors; the Black Weekly and National Media; John Blassingame, Publisher, Hype Hair and President, New Day Associates; Janell Agyeman, Literary Agent; and Shamboosie for his unwavering dedication to teach Black Women everything they need to know about their hair.

Appendix A

Let's Talk it Over:
Questions and Answers

Q. How often should I shampoo and condition my daughter's hair?
A. Contrary to popular belief, shampooing and conditioning should occur as often as possible. The more you shampoo and condition, the better it is for your hair, but remember that the use of good quality products will make the difference. When it comes to newborns, no conditioners are required. The baby care products will take care of the rest.

Q. Are Kiddie Perms safe?
A. They are safe, as long as they are not harsh chemicals, such as the No Lye Relaxer. *Please don't put that stuff in your child's hair.* Look for the labels that say Conditioning Lye Relaxer. Select Mild or Regular strength, then use as directed.

Q. Will rubber bands and hair ornaments damage my child's hair?
A. Rubber bands that are wrapped too tightly can cause hair breakage. Use coated rubber bands that are ¼ inch wide and that leave enough stretching ability, so they can be removed easily.

Q. Is styling gel safe to use in my daughter's hair?
A. Yes, by all means. The ones recommended in this book will dry soft, not hard or flaky.

Q. My daughter wants to get extensions. At what age is this O.K.?
A. I suggest that you take the proper steps to insure that her own hair will grow long and healthy. This is possible if you use good Hair Care Products and methods. If you must resort to extensions, any age after three years is okay, but you must take proper care of them and make sure they're not too tight. The extensions should be removed, and the hair should be gently relaxed every six to eight weeks. Then have the extensions put back in. This is a temporary fix, and it should always be thought of this way.

187

Q. Are you familiar with the Shea Butter/Jojoba Oil combination for babies' hair?

A. I have heard from some Moms that Shea Butter is a good product and that it works well. I am told that the Shea Butter/Jojoba Oil combination works well to soften the hair and add needed moisture. I sent my daughter a special formula of Shea Butter to treat her daughter's extremely dry skin, and it worked quite well. Shea Butter can be found in most health food stores, and it has become one of the most popular new products at all of the big hair shows. Jojoba oil is an ingredient found in many of the finest hair care products. It acts as a moisturizer and it is very good for the hair. Shea Butter/Jojoba Oil make a really good combination.

Q. I was told it is okay to relax my hair every four weeks. How often should my retouch be done?

A. The recommended time for a retouch is every six to eight weeks, not four, five or nine weeks, or the hair could start to break at the *line of demarcation*, which is where the new growth and the relaxed hair meet. The recommended time is determined by the speed at which your hair grows. Waiting at least six weeks gives you the needed time to condition the hair, which will keep it strong and prepare it to receive each *retouch*. A retouch means the new growth that needs to be relaxed. An important thing to remember is that the chemical should ONLY be applied to your new growth and not combed through the rest of your hair.

Q. What is the chemical difference between the curl and the relaxer?

A. Sodium or lye relaxer is designed to relax the hair by permanently removing those sometimes very tight, kinky curls. It is the most potent hair care product on the market.

The curl, on the other hand, is designed for rearranging the curl pattern in the hair. The bonds that form the natural curl in your hair, are temporarily rearranged, and the bonds that cause the natural curl to be unmovable or locked in are temporarily disconnected from each other. The hair is then wrapped around perm rods of different sizes to form the newly rearranged curls, which will be the size of the rods used. When the hair is neutralized, the bonds that cause the curls to be locked in are reconnected, and the new curl becomes permanent.

If you are wearing the curl, it is recommended that you not straighten your hair with a lye relaxer. If you do, you will lose a lot of hair. Also, it is not possible to put a curl over a lye relaxer, because the lye in the hair has destroyed all of the bonds that are needed to form the new curl.

Although the curl, which is made of ammonium thioglycolate, is also designed to straighten or relax the hair, it is not designed to be worn in a dry set or style for long periods of time. This also means you cannot blow-dry and style hair that is meant to be worn as a curl for more than two to three days. You must shampoo and condition the hair and return to the curly style after two or three days, or the hair will begin to shed by the handful. This is why you are always told to keep moisture in your curl. By moisture I mean softness, not wetness.

Q. Does Super strength mean it is a very strong relaxer.
A. There is very little difference in strength of "super," "regular," and "mild" relaxers. If they are conditioning lye relaxers, you should know that all three chemicals are mild enough, and the sodium content, the lye, is small enough to sustain the presence of the conditioners within the formula. A very strong relaxer would do just the opposite. It would eat away those conditioners. Often clients are uncomfortable with the term "super." So when I have to refer to a "super" relaxer in the salon and in their presence, I refer to it as a "number three."

The term "super" simply means for coarse or resistant hair, which is many times large in diameter. It DOES NOT mean strong. "Regular" relaxer is for a medium texture of hair, which is average in diameter, and it is the most widely-used of the three because most people do not have a coarse texture of hair. The "mild" relaxer is for color-treated or fine hair, and for hair that is in poor condition.

It is possible for all three textures of hair to be resistant, depending upon the texture of the hair and the ethnicity of the client. Do not assume that only black people have over-curly or kinky hair and are the only users of chemical relaxers. Women of other races use relaxers as well.

Q. I have been getting my hair relaxed for quite some time, and the hair in my nape area is very short and thinning out in places. Can you tell me why this is happening and how to stop the breakage?
A. This is one of the most serious, but common, problems I deal with in the salon. The reason for the breakage is the towel which was draped around the neck during a relaxer process. The towel should always be replaced with a clean one, once all of the relaxer is rinsed from the hair. In fact, everything that the relaxer has touched should be cleaned once the hair is rinsed and before the hair is neutralized. All combs, the shampoo bowl and the draining cup, any brushes or towels should be cleaned. Why? To avoid the possibility of any relaxer getting back into the hair, even the least little bit.

189

Residuals from the relaxer remain in the towel, although the hair has been rinsed, neutralized, conditioned, blown dry, curled and styled. The relaxer is still in the hair, working long after you leave the salon. Those residuals from the chemical left in the towel are fed back into the hair in the nape area, and still working while you are minding your own business at home. The solution is simple. Be sure that your stylist changes the towel.

Q. My stylist relaxed my hair last week and it looked good until I shampooed and conditioned my hair. A few days later, my hair was just as curly as if it had not been relaxed. What happened?
A. One of two things happened. First, if the chemical did not remain on the hair long enough to relax it, the hair would revert. Most of the time this is not the case. The other reason is one that is discussed many times in this book. It is possible that a no-lye relaxer was used in your hair. Sometimes, the use of this chemical will not completely straighten the hair. When this happens, some curl remains in the hair.

The no-lye relaxer locks the remaining curl in the hair, and nothing will remove it. The hair will appear straight while it's being relaxed, but as soon as it is shampooed, the curl returns. You must continue getting your hair relaxed every six to eight weeks, and use a quality conditioning lye relaxer. It leaves the hair softer with more moisture.

Q. Every time my hair is relaxed it becomes hard to manage. It will not hold curls, appears thinner, lifeless, and has no body. What is a girl to do?
A. The relaxer causes the hair strands to become smaller in diameter, which is the reason the relaxer should never be combed through the hair. A couple of days after the relaxer service, the cuticle layer, or the outer layer of the hair will open, and the hair will become larger in diameter. This will give a fuller look to your hair, and managing and styling the hair will be easier.

Q. Is it okay to use a lye relaxer over a no-lye relaxer?
A. Yes. You should know by now how I feel about the no-lye relaxer. Using a lye relaxer over a no-lye, if it is a high quality conditioning relaxer, could be one of the best things for your hair, because it will improve the overall condition of your hair. This is one way to make the transition from the no-lye to the lye relaxer. Some shedding may occur, however, this is normal. Condition the hair well, and this problem should clear up in a few days.

190

On the other hand, crossing a no-lye relaxer over a lye relaxer is not a good idea, regardless of the quality of the no lye relaxer. If you are not wearing a Conditioning Lye Relaxer, get one, and stay with it.

If you are using a lye relaxer, but are having a problem with burning during the application, introduce your stylist to System #1. It is a "no burn" technique that will work every time.

Q. Please give me some tips on how to manage and care for my hair at home. I have worn a relaxer for many years.

A. Buy the best quality shampoo and conditioner available. Shampoo and condition at least once a week, or every four days, for two months, then once a week for life. Do a treatment after every chemical service. *Conditioning the hair is an absolute must!* Mix a leave-in conditioner with some setting lotion, and spray in your hair. Detangle, dry the hair, and use a hairdressing. The hair should have just enough shine to create a healthy appearance. Then set or curl the hair, and style as usual.

Q. Can I relax my hair and permanently color my hair in the same day?

A. No! Wait at least a week, and do one or two shampoo and conditioning treatments before coloring the hair. If you desire to color, and absolutely must do a relaxer at the same time, have it done professionally. Your hairdresser should do the relaxer first, as it is the harsher of the two chemicals. From this point on, the way you care for your hair will have to change. The conditioner should be one with *more protein* and *less moisture*. The conditioner should be applied every four days, for four to six weeks, then once per week with no exceptions.

Q. I am so tired of wearing the curl. How can I safely grow out of it?

A. This is one of the hardest things to do. After wearing a curl for a long period of time, the hair will become very soft and very weak. The changes that the chemical has caused in the hair cannot be reversed. The best you can do is to settle for a short haircut. I don't suggest you cut all the hair off and start over. However, eventually all of the chemically treated hair will go, if not by cutting it off, the hair will probably fall out on its own. Putting a relaxer in this hair could possibly speed up the breakage process. This is your only way out of the curl, but the good news is your hair should grow back in about 24 to 36 months.

If you choose to get a relaxer after a curl, treat the hair every three days for about four weeks with a protein conditioner to make the hair as strong as possible. Then use a mild conditioning lye relaxer, and have it applied to the new growth only. Do not smooth or allow the chemical to remain in the hair too long. You only want to remove about 60 percent of the curl in the new growth. Continue with treatments, and relax the hair every six weeks in the same manner until you have grown one-and-a half to two inches of new hair.

Remember, you could possibly lose some hair as you are making the transition, but the hair would do the same thing if you did not make the transition and discontinue using the curl. Treat the hair as if it is still a curl, with activators and moisturizers but don't over do it. Get a fresh haircut and keep the ends trimmed.

You may blow dry the hair and go straight for two or three days at a time, but you must shampoo, condition and return to the curl. If you decide to go straight and stay straight, use a good hairdressing to help keep the hair soft. Whatever you do, DO NOT hot press your new growth for this is the quickest way to go bald. Good Luck.

Q. What is meant by the term "overlapping"?
A. If I could curb this one practice (overlapping), I could save many women a lot of their hair. This is very important. Each time you return for a retouch on haircolor, the curl, highlights or relaxer, it is because you have new growth, possibly one-half to four inches. The correct way to apply product for a retouch in any of these situations is apply to the new growth only. The part of the hair shaft where the new growth meets with the previous chemically treated hair is called the *line of demarcation*.

Any time the chemical is applied to both the new growth and the chemically treated hair in the same and a single application, it is called *overlapping*, and it is never a good idea. There is always a chance of overlapping, especially when chemically relaxing the hair. It is almost impossible not to. The problem is that most people go too far by *combing* the chemical through all of the hair. This is a point I have tried very hard to stress in teaching haircare professionals over the years. However, many stylists disregard this most important application technique.

Think of it this way. There is absolutely no need to relax, color, highlight, or perm hair that has already received these services. The prevention of overlapping is the only way to protect the previously chemically treated hair, thus preventing damage to that hair. This is ironic because every hair care professional and Basic Cosmetology student is taught to do it this way, yet many do not.

Q. I have been using a semi permanent haircolor to cover my gray, and as soon as I shampoo, the gray hair is back. I am afraid to use permanent haircolor. What can I do to cover my gray?

A. There are many ways to cover, blend or color gray hair that will last much longer.

One way is called long lasting semi-permanent haircolor and another is called permanent haircolor, but be sure to use a low volume developer. You are not changing the color of your hair but just covering the gray, and a ten volume developer will do the job in as little as ten minutes. Add two ounces of shampoo to the formula to weaken the developer even more and lessen its effect on the hair. You only want to *deposit* color, which happens quickly. These formulas are very mild and safe for your hair. They also condition as they color the hair, and you can relax the hair safely while using these haircoloring formulas.

Q. Every time I comb my hair, I see a lot of hair in the comb and all over the place. What can I do to stop the breakage?

A. Many times we go too long without a shampoo and a very good conditioner. The hair must be fed regularly, the same way we must be fed. Imagine not eating for weeks, or months at a time. What do you think would happen to you? You would "fall out."

The same thing happens to your hair. Your hair must be fed, on time, at least once a week. To stop breakage, use a *deep penetrating protein conditioning treatment*, the best quality you can buy, and follow it with a *crème conditioner*. Condition every four days for thirty days, then once a week.

Q. My stylist has been using products on my hair that were not made for black hair, is this okay?

A. Do not select your hair care products on the basis of whether they were made by a white or black hair product company. A good conditioner will work regardless of who makes it. The reality is there are more good white hair care products on the market than there are good black hair care products, because white companies have been making good hair care products for a longer period of time. It takes identically the same raw materials to make a good product, no matter who makes it.

My hope is that after you read this book, you will remove the terms *black* and *white* from the whole idea of purchasing good products for your hair. The deciding factor should be whether the product works or not. If the product works, keep using it regardless of who makes it.

Never use a hair care product just because you like it or because it smells good, or because it feels good. Listen to expert advice, and buy only the best products for your hair, and use them on a regular basis. The better the quality of the product, the better the job the product will do. The better condition your hair is in, the more beautiful, you will look and feel.

Q. Every time I shampoo my curl, it takes days to get my hair to look good again. Is there anything you can tell me that will help?
A. The solution is very simple. Some people have used this problem as an excuse to not shampoo and condition their hair. Don't make the same mistake. There is no excuse for neglecting the care of your hair. Your hair should look good and feel nice and soft the same day you shampoo and treat your hair. It is so important to shampoo and condition the curl once a week with a good conditioner. These tips will work every time, even after a fresh new curl. This is how we do it.

Make sure your stylist uses an activator and a moisturizer before you leave the salon.

When you get home, use your activator and moisturizer every thirty minutes for two hours. Apply each time as if it is the first application.

The hair can only hold so much of the product at one time, so even if you pile it on, all that the hair will not receive will simply dry up before the hair can absorb it. After the fourth application, the hair will look as good as it did before the shampoo and conditioner. Your problem is you have been putting too much time between the replenishing applications, causing the hair to dry out completely before the next application. This is the reason it seems to take days to get the hair to look good. Putting the activator and moisturizer in every thirty minutes for the first two hours will fill the hair with all the moisture it needs before it has a chance to dry out, and your hair will be soft to the touch, but not wet.

Q. I have gray hair, but I'm having trouble getting out "the yellow." What causes the hair to turn yellow?
A. White hair, like anything else that is white, gets dirty. The problem could be due to a buildup of hair care product, hot curling too often, or not shampooing often enough with a shampoo designed for cleaning gray hair. In studying haircolor, we learn that violet is the color that will neutralize yellow. With this in mind, look for a shampoo that is designed for this purpose. It will have violet in its formula. Be sure to read everything on the label before applying to the hair, and use as directed.

194

Shampoo and condition your hair every four days, until "you wonder where the yellow went." There are many shampoos designed to neutralize yellow on the market, so help should be easy to find.

Clairol has a complete line of haircolor designed especially for gray hair. You can cover your gray, make it darker, and even neutralize the yellow. I'm sure there is a shade to match your haircolor exactly.

Q. Why are so many women suffering from dry hair?
The biggest reason of all is the use of no-lye relaxer. Other reasons are not conditioning properly, lack of moisture, permanently coloring the hair at home, the use of cheap products, and the list goes on. The dryness has taken out all of their hair, leaving many women of color believing that the only way to have long, flowing, beautiful hair is to resort to braiding, weaving, locs, wigs and an assortment of other hair extension possibilities. Switching to a natural hairstyle is a wonderful idea, but many of the reasons for switching are not so wonderful.

Q. There seems to be an overwhelming lack of understanding about hair care problems in general. Why?
A. The answer is simple. There is a lack of education. Most women simply don't know what to do. They have "tried this" and they have "tried that," and they have never been satisfied. However, they can learn how to properly care for their hair. They usually feel that chemicals are the biggest cause of Hair Care Problems, but there are others reasons. The blame is to be placed on lack of knowledge and not on the products. It is simply a "learn it" (proper haircare) or "lose it" (your hair), proposition. Unfortunately, many women have lost a lot of hair.

Q. Why are so many of women so trusting of the opinions of so many people, their friends, Hair Care Companies and even hair care professionals?
A. For so long, the black woman has had so many concerns and no real answers. She has been confused about what to do next. You can find the answers here, I promise.

Q. Why are women trying so many unproven products on their hair and their children's hair?
A. It's really crazy. It's because of a lack of knowledge or that they simply don't know any better.

Q. Why do so many believe they can just stop using chemicals, buy some natural hair products, use them, and everything will be just fine?
A. The chemicals in the hair will not "just go away," and to just stop the use is a very dangerous thing to do. The truth of the matter is that if she stops

using chemicals, she will lose hair, and a lot of it. Ridding the hair of chemicals takes some time, about two years, to grow the hair and cut the chemically treated hair off. Even with use of the best shampoos and conditioners during this period, there is still a real chance of some hair loss. However, if the hair is already very short, the transition will be much easier.

Q. What are some examples of semi-permanent haircolor?
Clairol's Beautiful Browns, Jazzing, and colored mousses, are some examples of semi-permanent haircolor that simply coat the hair shaft or penetrate slightly. When applied properly they can last 2 to 4 shampoos. When temporary, semi-permanent and long lasting semi-permanent haircolor are mixed with 10-volume peroxide, they will last up to 24 shampoos, if you shampoo and condition your hair often.

Q. What should you consider when choosing a haircolor?
Always consider these factors:
- The color presently in the hair
- Your natural shade
- Your skin tone
- Your eye color
- Your age
- Your occupation
- Your life style
- The current condition of your hair

Q. What are some of the better shades for women of color?
Gold, Warm Browns, Blond and Auburn shades, colors containing some Reds, Real Reds, Dark Brown, Black, and Blue Black are well-suited to brown skin tones. To be honest, you can wear *any* color hair you want from, black to blond, but keep it warm.

Q. Curls, haircolor, relaxers, which will do the most damage?
When these products are used as directed, the level of change and damage to your hair texture will be minimal, in most cases, about the same for all three. Significant damage is caused by misuse or by error in formulation, application, or processing time.

Q. Should I color my gray, and if so, what is the best way?
Yes, color it, if you desire. If the gray is greater than 50% and you are staying with your natural shade, use a permanent haircolor with 20-volume developer for the best results. If the gray is less than 25%, use a long lasting semi-permanent haircolor with a 10-volume developer.

There are also products available for blending gray, or enhancing your gray hair for beautiful hair if you like gray hair. Included in this book is a list of recommended products that address your various haircolor cares. Available also is a list of products that can be used to keep your gray hair looking vibrant and healthy. Remember the better quality of the product, the better the results.

Q. Will the amount and length of my hair make a difference when coloring?
Yes. Color works best when the hair is saturated with the product. This means that as much as 2 bottles of haircolor, 4 ounces may be needed to do the job. This will become 8 full ounces when mixed with 4 ounces of developer, but you should never need any more than 4 ounces. When the hair is 6 to 8 inches long or less, 2 ounces of color and 2 ounces of developer will do just fine.

If the hair is long, remember that the ends of the hair have been around longer and are very porous. When going darker than your natural color, the ends will grab more color and end up darker than the rest of the hair. Therefore, the new growth, midshaft, and the ends will have to be handled separately. If you have had color before and are getting a retouch, you will need 2 different formulas, one permanent color for the new growth, and the other a semi-permanent color to refresh the color of the midshaft and ends of your hair. The ends are porous and they will absorb color faster. It is best to see a professional.

Q. Should I shampoo my hair before I color it?
It depends on the type of color you are using. It is okay to shampoo if you are using temporary, semi, semi-permanent or a long lasting semi-permanent haircolor, but delay conditioning until you finish coloring the hair. If the hair is oily or there is a build-up on the hair shaft, a clarifying shampoo, which is designed specifically for deep cleansing, may be needed. However, do not shampoo your hair if you are using a permanent haircolor, because a developer is part of the formula, and it should only be applied to dry hair. Remember to be very gentle when massaging the scalp. Allow a few days between the shampoo and the use of permanent haircolor. Always read the directions completely before you start the application. You should do the same with every hair care product you intend to use on your hair.

Q. I have heard so much about the strand test, why is it important?
This is one of the most important things you can do before coloring, because it is the surest way to know the end result before you color your hair. If you were to use the same color as a friend, your color, in most cases, would turn out a different color than your friend's.

The reason is that no two people have the same natural color hair. The only time the hair will turn out the same, is if you going darker. Remember, there are some hidden colors in your hair that will surprise you. These are called "contributing pigments." Do a strand test to determine the appropriate timing to predict an accurate result.

Q. Will my hair type (straight, curly, dry or oily, coarse or fine) change the time it will take to color my hair?
Yes. Coarse hair will take longer for the color to penetrate. With medium and fine hair it is much faster. Whether the hair is straight, curly or oily, makes no difference.

Q. What is meant by double processing?
If the color you desire requires lifting your natural color 2 or 3 shades lighter, toning to achieve the desired shade is called "a double process." In addition, anytime there is a chemical already in the hair, the addition of another chemical is "double processing." If you have three chemicals in the hair this is called "triple processing." Triple processing is never recommended.

First the hair is lightened with a bleach or lightener. The toner is applied to give the hair its desired shade. This process will require a professional because the chosen toner must have the exact base color, which is found on every bottle of permanent haircolor. It is best to consult a professional colorist who understands how to choose and use the base color.

Appendix B

Author Recommendations for Your Hair Care Maintenance

Home Maintenance Prescriptions from Dudley Products

Product Description

By using the products recommended here, you can create a personalized home care maintenance regime especially for your hair type and special needs.

- ❑ **Hair Rebuilder** is a penetrating conditioner for badly damaged hair.

- ❑ **Moisturizing Conditioner** is high in Vitamin A and other minerals needed to moisturize the hair.

- ❑ **Cream Protein** is a moisturizer that strengthens, softens and restores moisture in the hair shaft.

- ❑ **The Shampoo** is a versatile, acid-balanced shampoo that removes oil and residue from the hair.

- ❑ **Deluxe Shampoo** is an acid-balanced, conditioning shampoo that greatly improves the quality and texture of natural, relaxed, bleached and color-treated hair.

- ❑ **Dandruff Shampoo** is a medicated, conditioning shampoo that is mild on the scalp, eliminates dandruff and stops minor scalp irritation and itching.

- ❑ **Fantastic Body Setting Lotion** is a versatile styling lotion designed to create body, radiant sheen and firm hold for wet setting, sculpturing, and blow-drying.

- ❑ **Crème Press** is a light, creamy oil blend designed to coat and protect the hair from the damaging effects of excessive thermal or blow-drying heat.

- ❑ **Total Control Styling Spray** is a protein-enriched styling spray that lets you sculpt, spike, shape, mold and lock in style definition.

- ❑ **PCA Moisture Retainer** is a concentrated, leave-in moisturizing hair dressing designed to restore the hair's natural oils and moisture.

- ❑ **Vitamin AD & E Hair and Scalp Conditioner** is an extra light oil designed to lubricate the scalp and soften the hair by supplementing the scalp's natural oils.

- ❑ **Scalp Special** is a light hair and scalp oil that helps control itchy scalp.

Phone: 1-800-334-4150
Website: www.dudleyq.com

"Feed Your Hair"
Product Description

Nexxus conditioners will make your hair strong, shiny, bouncy, and beautiful. Nexxus is environmentally friendly and never tested on animals. These are a few of Shamboosie's recommendations:

- ❑ KerapHix Creme Reconstructor

  Restructuring Conditioner for Stressed Hair. Rebuilder, Reconditioner
  Strengthens dry, brittle hair; keratin protein reinforces hair integrity prior to chemical services; corrects heat damage from thermal appliances; mends split ends. Usage: 1-2 times per week.

- ❑ Humectress Moisturizing Conditioner

  Rehydrator, Moisture Rebalancer. Smoothes, soothes and relieves dry, frizzy hair; contains sunscreen and protects against thermal appliances. Usage: daily, as needed.

❑ Aloe Rid Clarifying Treatment

Detoxifier, Build-up Remover, Purifier. Removes build-up from minerals, chlorine, fluoride, medication, styling products, pool and spa water. Usage: 1-2 times per week, as needed, and prior to all chemical services.

❑ Headress Leave-in Conditioner

Hairdressing Pomade, Bodifier, Detangler, Ultra lightweight; detangles; bodifies with vitamin B5; great thermal protectant and cutting/wrapping lotion. Usage: daily, as needed.

❑ Vita Tress Biotin Creme

Effective scalp treatment specifically formulated for problems related to fragile, thinning hair. Usage: nightly.

❑ Emergencee Polymeric Reconstructor

Structural Modifier, Reconditioner, Restructuring Conditioner Restructures cuticle and inner cortex of hopelessly damaged hair; acidifies; reconstructs and strengthens stressed hair; stops breakage and prepares hair to accept chemical services. Usage: 1 time per week, as needed.

❑ Botanoil Treatment Shampoo

Treatment for Stressed or Chemically Processed Hair Strengthens, improves elasticity, pliability; replenishes essential fatty acids.

❑ Aloe Rid Clarifying Shampoo

Detoxifier, Build-up Remover, Purifier, Alternative Shampoo Clarifies internal and external hair shaft; removes environmental pollutants, medication, pool and spa chemicals, minerals and styling product build-up.

❑ Diametress Hair Thickening Shampoo

Bodifier, Volumizer, Texturizer. Adds body and fullness; increases strength, elasticity and diameter of hair shaft.

❑ Vita Tress Biotin Shampoo

Revitalizer, Energizer, Nourisher. Removes sebum on scalp; infuses nutrients into hair and scalp; strengthens and fortifies fine, thin, fragile hair.

Nexxus guarantees satisfaction on all genuine Nexxus Products purchased at hairstyling salons. Money will be refunded upon return of product and receipt to the salon of purchase. Exchanges can be made at any salon retailing the Nexxus line upon presentation of product.

Website: www.nexxus.com

Safety Issues

Understanding haircolor was discussed in Chapter 8. However, some of the safety issues with regard to haircolor will be addressed here. We will also talk about concerns and precautions that should be followed in other areas of hair care.

Are haircoloring products safe to use on human hair? This is a very important question. For some time now the Food and Drug Administration (FDA) has been considering a proposal to change the way haircolor is made. The matter has become complicated because some studies have linked haircoloring with an increased risk of contracting certain cancers. There are other studies that do not support those findings, making this issue a controversial one. Pre-market testing for the safety of most haircolor is less strenuous than those of other cosmetic color additives. The decision to use permanent haircolor and its safe is mostly left up to the consumer.

I have never met anyone who has had any problems resulting from the use of haircolor, with the exception of an occasional skin reaction, which can easily be eliminated by following certain safety precautions. Information concerning these precautions and proper application methods for haircolor can be found in "The Color of Hair."

The FDA oversees the safety of all cosmetics sold in the United States, and it can disallow the sale of any cosmetic found to be harmful, except most hair dyes. This provision of the FDA can and will seek removal of a cosmetic from the market if it is shown to be harmful under conditions of use. Hair coloring made from coal tar was given special exemption from bans when the act was passed many years ago. The laws pertaining to the ingredient found in the coal tar haircolors that prompted an allergic reaction in some sus ceptible individuals has not changed much over the years. Mo hair dyes in use today derive their ingredients from petroleum sources, but have been considered coal tar dyes by the FDA because they contain some of the same compounds found in older permanent haircolors.

Fearing that the FDA would ban the sale of hair dyes because some users might develop allergic reactions, the industry successfully lobbied before the act passed to get coal tar hair dyes exempted from the provisions. Therefore, it was decided that a consumer's advisory be required, in the form of a warning label on every package, stating that the product can cause skin irritation in certain allergic individuals. If you are already using permanent haircolor, enjoy it. If you are not, but desire to, trust your stylist and this book. Find a good colorist and depend on that colorist to do the best job when coloring your hair.

Using Haircolor During Pregnancy

If you are concerned about the safety of having your hair colored while pregnant, allow me to say this. Certain studies have attempted to identify the risk of various cancers to people that use permanent haircolor by estimating the dissimilarities in frequency of cancer in people who use permanent haircolor and those who do not. There is no proof that use of haircolor is harmful to pregnant women.

The same studies failed to consider the effects of other causes of cancer such as cigarette smoking, when comparing users and non-users. The findings to date are inconclusive. To simplify, there is no basis to say that haircolor poses a definitive risk of cancer.

Using Chemical Relaxer During Pregnancy

f you were using chemical relaxers before pregnancy, you still
ed to have your hair relaxed every 6 to 8 weeks. The concerns
should have with a chemical relaxer are constant… scalp
hair breakage, and dryness. If you are pregnant, the only
oblem you may have is some discomfort when laying back
hampoo chair for a long period of time. Other than that, you
't have any concerns about having your hair relaxed while
regnant. Relax, it's okay.

Other Precautions

Never color your eyebrows or eyelashes, and don't allow it to be done in the salon. An allergic reaction to the haircolor could prompt swelling, inflammation, and susceptibility to infection in the sensitive eye area. Such reactions could severely harm the eyes and even cause blindness. Improper application or an accidental spilling of the color into the eye could cause permanent damage. The FDA prohibits the sale or use of haircolor for eyelash and eyebrow tinting or coloring even in beauty salons. It's the law.

Researchers continue to study the cancer-causing potential of hair dye ingredients, and the FDA continues to monitor the findings of this research. Always exercise caution when selecting and using any haircoloring product.

If you use permanent haircolor follow these safety precautions:

❑ Be sure to do a patch test for allergic reactions before applying the dye to your hair.

❑ Wear gloves when applying hair dye.

❑ Do not leave the dye on any longer than necessary.

❑ Rinse scalp thoroughly with water after use.

❑ Follow directions on the label carefully.

❑ Never mix different hair dye products, because you can induce potentially harmful reactions (and you could produce really unappealing haircolor).

Almost all hair dye products include instructions for conducting a patch test, and it is important to perform the test every time you dye your hair. Every salon should require a patch test before performing a color service, and the client should insist that a patch test be done.

To test at home, put a dab of hair dye behind your ear, and don't wash it off for two days. If no itching, burning, redness or other signs of allergic reaction develop at the test spot, you can be relatively sure that you won't develop a reaction to the coloring product when applied to your hair. If you do react to the patch test, perform the same test with different brands or colors until you find one to which you are not allergic. They are *not* all the same.

Use Caution with Aerosol Hairspray Products

Care should always be taken when using aerosol hairspray products. It is very easy for these products to catch fire if exposed to an open flame, a lit cigarette, the striking of matches or lighters, or the stove that is used for heating curling irons.

Keep aerosol product containers away from children. A match and an aerosol container can become an instant torch in the hands of a child. Aerosol product hairspray fires are particularly dangerous because the product is used in the process of hair care services and used mostly around the head. If human hair catches fire, it can burn so fast that it could result in complete baldness in a matter of seconds. Others nearby may also be subject to injury. I once witnessed such a tragedy, and I can tell you it was very frightening.

Warnings are found on the labels and instructions on how these products should be used. Avoid heat, fire, and smoking during use until sprayed hair is fully dry and all of the residuals are no longer airborne. An FDA warning was prompted by recent reports of injuries and deaths resulting from aerosol hairspray-related fires.

As with many aerosol cosmetic and household products, the flammability of most aerosol sprays is attributable to the use of hydrocarbon propellants in combination with SD alcohol 40 solvent. This mixture has been widely used to replace chlorofluorocarbons CFCs, which were banned from aerosol propellant use in the United States in 1978 because of environmental concerns.

The FDA is exploring ways to enhance the effectiveness of label warnings. The agency is also looking into new approaches for heightening consumer awareness of hairspray-related fire hazards to protect the public health.

The Glossary

Alkaline Perm

A permanent wave product with a pH from 7.5 to 9.5. It is stronger, producing a more firm, springy curl. The term usually refers to the product used to put curl in white hair.

Ammonia

The substance in permanent haircolor, which causes the developer to lighten the hair while at the same time enabling the color to be deposited into the hair, thereby changing the color of the hair. *Ammonia* is an alkaline found in haircolor, and is that ingredient which causes hair to become porous during the coloring process. When selecting a haircolor, choose one that is ammonia-free.

Ammonium Thioglycolate

Also known as (Thio) or (The Curl). It is an active chemical ingredient in permanent waves and ethnic curly perm products.

Basing Cream

A protective oily cream that is applied to the scalp, ears, and neck before applying a lye relaxer, and sometimes a curl product to minimize the skin irritation when it comes into contact with the chemical. It is important to choose one made for this purpose.

Bonding

Weaves, braids and extensions are all methods of temporarily adding and attaching wefts, locks or small sections of synthetic and human hair. Bonding holds them in place.

Bonds of the Hair   The chemical makeup of the hair. There are *disulfide bonds* that keep the hair in its curly position. The *hydrogen bonds* are the weakest of the lot. Getting control of these bonds is easy. They control the polypeptide chain which holds the hair in a straight position. The *saline bonds* are broken very quickly after the chemical is applied to the hair, with just a little manipulation by the hand and comb.

Bleach or Bleaching   A Lightener which comes in powder, cream, or gel form. Bleach chemically strips so much more than just color from the hair. In many cases, it leaves black hair lifeless. It is very dangerous to apply other chemicals, such as relaxers, and thio perms, on top of bleach. Bleaching should *never* be done at home. In fact, I do not recommend bleaching at all. There are many other safer ways to lighten hair.

Clarifying Shampoo   Used to remove most any type buildup on the hair. It contains a strong detergent base for deep cleaning.

Color Remover   Designed for removing unwanted artificial haircolor. There are separate color removers for permanent and semi-permanent haircolor.

Coolness of haircolor   *Blue, green* and *violet*-base tones in permanent haircolor are referred to as *cool*. Their job is to enhance or neutralize unwanted tones when coloring hair.

Curl Activator   A cream created to add moisture or softness to the hair and it activates the new curl. The absence of this product will leave the hair dry with an appearance of natural, kinky hair.

Curl Moisturizer   A maintenance product for chemically curled hair, used to soften, moisturize, and "revive" the curl.

Dandruff   A white flaky buildup of dead skin cells found on an oily scalp or a dry scalp, which means the flakes can be dry or oily.

Elasticity	The hair's ability to stretch without breaking and return to its original shape. It is very difficult to see with the naked eye, which is the reason it should be avoided at all cost. It will happen easily if you comb the hair when there are chemicals in the hair or when the hair is wet. The *elasticity* determines how well the hair will hold curl, which is an important factor in choosing the correct perms, type of haircolor and relaxers.
Hair Follicle	The opening in the scalp through which a single strand of hair grows.
Henna	This is an ancient Egyptian vegetable dye in powder form, which gives the hair reddish tones. Its name is derived from the plant from which it is made. *Henna* is metallic in nature, which means that once it is applied to the hair, this product will block any application of an ammonia/peroxide base haircolor.
Hydrogen Peroxide	A liquid or cream chemical *developer*. When mixed with permanent haircolor, it lifts the natural pigmentation or color of the hair, at the same time, preparing the hair for the deposit of the new color. It also activates the lifting ingredient of powder, gel and cream lightners.
Hairdressing	A maintenance product that gives the hair a slight sheen or shine. The best hairdressing comes in the form of a light cream that conditions, moisturizes and leaves the hair soft and silky to the touch. *Hairdressing* can be used daily to give the hair a healthier appearance.
Grease	This product should be used lightly *on the scalp*, but *never on the hair*. In some cases it may be used to base the scalp, but only when designed for that purpose. *Grease* should never be used for "dressing the hair" because it is usually too oily.
Highlights	Strands of hair that are colored selectively creating a "streaked" effect.

Level System	All natural haircolors fall within 10 levels of shades, from black to lightest blond. Hair color manufacturers use a *level system* to chart their many different shades and colors, from *warmest* brown, red and gold, to the *coolest* ash shades.
Lye	The chemical ingredient used to formulate *sodium hydroxide* relaxers. When formulated with a conditioner, it becomes the best method of relaxing human hair (*lye* as opposed to "*no-lye*").
Low Lights	After the hair has received as many highlights as possible, an opposite process of toning some strands of hair is referred to as *low lighting*. Usually haircolors mixed with 10-volume developer or semi-permanent haircolors are used for this purpose. The same effect can be used to create soft or subtle *highlights* in black hair by breaking the base color of some strands of hair around the face. Use only a 10 volume developer.
Melanin	The pigment that makes up hair's natural color. There are two types — Eumelanin makes the dark or black pigment in hair, and Pheomelanin, makes the red/yellow pigment in hair. A mixture of the two is called Mixed Melanin. If the hair has no color, it has no melanin.
Metallic Dye	Hair color that comes from metallic salts and from lead.
Neutralizer	The chemical applied at the end of a curl or relaxer to completely stop the chemical process and return the hair to its normal pH level. Sold in clear liquid, cream, lotion and shampoo form.
Neutralizing Shampoo	This product is the only kind of shampoo to use when doing a chemical relaxer service. It is the only thing that will stop the relaxer from working.

No-Lye Relaxer

The common term for every chemical used to relax hair that **does not** contain *sodium hydroxide* as its active chemical ingredient. The *calcium hydroxide relaxer* (the "BALD" faced "LYE") is by far the most dangerous, but the most widely-used, relaxer on the market today. Even if you use it only one time, you could lose all of your hair, so stay away from this one. It is a very different product from the sodium hydroxide relaxer. Some others contain Ammonium Thioglycolate, Lithium Hydroxide and Potassium Hydroxide.

Porosity

The hair's ability to absorb moisture. When the hair is slightly porous, it is soft or moist, allowing chemical relaxer, haircolor and conditioners to ease their way through the cuticle layer, into the cortex layer of the hair. The no-lye relaxer restricts the hair's ability to absorb moisture by actually "locking it out." This causes the hair to be very dry and promotes the possibility of breakage.

Protein

A complex organic compound that contains amino acids as its basic structural units. It is found in all living tissue, skin, hair and nails. The hair is made up of about 98% protein, which is why there are many protein treatments designed to rebuild strength in hair that has lost its elasticity by adding protein to the cuticle and cortex layer of the hair. Most black Hair Care Products contain protein. If you always choose and use the best and highest quality of these products, they will give you the best chance for a healthy head of hair.

Remember, there is no substitute for quality Hair Care Products!

Over-Processed Hair	Hair that is dry, brittle, and damaged from the misuse of chemicals. Many women do their own chemical services at home without thorough knowledge of how the chemical process works. Also, most of the time people do not read or follow the instructions precisely. The hair can become over-processed from haircolor, perms, relaxers, and even conditioners. Some women have 2 to 4 chemicals in the hair at the same time, and each of these chemicals is applied and over-processed. This kind of damage could be also impossible to fix. Most of problems can be avoided by reading and following product instructions carefully.
Perm	The "relaxer" service used to be called "the perm," meaning permanently relaxed into a straight position. Today, "perm" refers to Thio, short for Ammonium Thioglycolate, which is "the curl" or "curly perm."
The "S" Pattern	When doing "a curl" the hair is wrapped around perm rods. A few of them must be unwrapped to check for a *well-defined wave pattern*, which is referred to as the "S" Pattern.
The "S" Curl	Hair that is relaxed 80% straight or less with a lye relaxer is referred to as the *"S"curl* and called a *texturizer.*
Sodium Hydroxide	A very high alkaline product used to permanently straighten hair. A *conditioning lye relaxer* is the very best way to relax the hair. Use only the very highest quality.
Setting Lotion	A medium hold product for hair that adds volume, shape and style and controls curls.
The pH Scale	The symbol for *Potential Hydrogen Concentration* - the degree of acidity or alkalinity of any water-based solution. A pH of 7 is neutral, on a scale from 0 (very acidic) to 14 (very alkaline). Human hair seems to thrive best at 4.5 to 6.5, a slightly acidic pH level. Permanent haircoloring is an alkaline chemical process, which temporarily raises the hair's pH to 10 or 11.

212

Processing Time

The amount of time haircolor, permanent waving solution or chemical relaxer remains on the hair before being rinsed out. The processing method is how the product works. Most perm products process at room temperature.

Resistant Hair

Hair that is very difficult to perm, chemically relax, or permanently color is called *resistant*. It means that the cuticle layer of the hair is very strong, and lies too flat and tightly against the hair shaft to allow moisture to enter. Many times the hair must be pre-softened to get the cuticle layer of the hair to open. This is also what will happen chemically when you use the no-lye relaxer. It will cause the hair to resist everything—conditioners, shampoo, water and even another relaxer.

Warm or warmth in haircolor

The colors *gold, orange* or *red-base* tones in permanent haircolor are referred to as *warm*. Their job is to enhance or neutralize unwanted tones when coloring hair.

Weave

A temporary way to add more hair to a person's real hair. Strands of human or synthetic hair are sewn, bonded or glued into place.

Weft

A lock of human or synthetic hair used for weaving, extensions and bonding. The weft holds the strands together.

Wrapping Lotion

A setting lotion that is used for molding smoothly wrapped sets. Any setting lotion will do the same thing.

Virgin Hair

Hair that has never been permed, colored, straightened or otherwise chemically treated.

About the Author

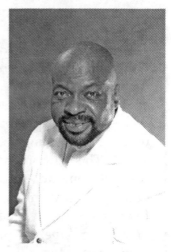

Shamboosie is a twenty-year veteran of the hair care industry. Shamboosie is a Color Master Consultant with Clairol Professional. His duties include promoting Clairol's line of relaxers and haircolors designed for women of color. He participates in hair shows and studio events around the country educating hairstylists about the use of the Clairol product line.

After completing his initial training in Cosmetology, Shamboosie became involved in sales, research, and testing of new products at Dudley Cosmetology University (DCU), in Kernersville, NC.

Later as an instructor of Advanced Techniques at DCU, Shamboosie trained hundred of hairstylists, and participated in artistic platform presentations. He can be seen in Dudley's Stylebook No. 3 instructing students in proper chemical application method.

Shamboosie continues to work in the hair care industry performing independent research, design, and development of ethnic hair care techniques, with a special concentration on problem-solving methods. Following his relocation to New Jersey, Shamboosie was recruited by one of the top salons, where he has continued to provide professional hair care services and training. He has recently received the Outstanding Service Award in recognition of his leadership, commitment, and dedication to the cosmetology industry.

Shamboosie and his wife, Marilyn, reside in Hackensack, NJ.

Disclaimer:

The entire substance of this book—all of the recommendations and advice offered —is the sole responsibility of the Author, and not that of Amber Books, the Publisher. For all chemical applications, such as permanent haircolor, chemical relaxers, curly perms and the like, the Author has stressed the necessity of seeking the advice of a qualified hair care professional. The Author's advice, recommended solutions to hair care problems and recommended products are of the highest quality, but will only work if the instructions of the Author are followed precisely. The Author strongly advises the reading of product labels (front and back) prior to purchase, and adherence to the product manufacturer's advice.

Enjoy your beautiful healthy hair; and God bless you and your family.

Shamboosie

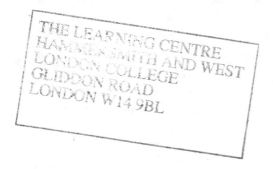

ORDER FORM

WWW.AMBERBOOKS.COM
African-American Self Help and Career Books

Fax Orders:	480-283-0991	Postal Orders: Send Checks & Money Orders to:
Telephone Orders:	1-866-566-3144	Amber Books Publishing
Online Orders: E-mail:	Amberbks@aol.com	1334 E. Chandler Blvd., Suite 5-D67 Phoenix, AZ 85048

_____ *Beautiful Black Hair: A Step-by-Step Instructional Guide*

_____ *How to Get Rich When You Ain't Got Nothing*

_____ *The African-American Travel Guide*

_____ *Suge Knight: The Rise, Fall, and Rise of Death Row Records*

_____ *The African-American Teenagers Guide to Personal Growth, Health, Safety, Sex and Survival*

_____ *Get That Cutie in Commercials, Televisions, Films & Videos*

_____ *Wake Up and Smell the Dollars! Whose Inner City is This Anyway?*

_____ *How to Own and Operate Your Home Day Care Business Successfully Without Going Nuts!*

_____ *The African-American Woman's Guide to Successful Make-up and Skin Care*

_____ *How to Play the Sports Recruiting Game and Get an Athletic Scholarship: The Handbook and Guide to Success for the African-American High School Student-Athlete*

_____ *Is Modeling for You? The Handbook and Guide for the Young Aspiring Black Model*

_____ *Wavy, Curly, Kinky: The African American Child's Hair Care Guide*

Name:_____

Company Name:_____

Address:_____

City:_____State:_____Zip:_____

Telephone: (_____) _____E-mail:_____

For Bulk Rates Call: **1-866-566-3144**   ## ORDER NOW

Beautiful Black Hair	$16.95	❑ Check ❑ Money Order ❑ Cashiers Check
How to Get Rich	$14.95	❑ Credit Card: ❑ MC ❑ Visa ❑ Amex ❑ Discover
Travel Guide	$14.95	CC#_____
Suge Knight	$21.95	
Teenagers Guide	$19.95	Expiration Date:_____
Cutie in Commercials	$16.95	
Wake Up & Smell the Dollars	$18.95	**Payable to:** Amber Books
Home Day Care	$12.95	1334 E. Chandler Blvd., Suite 5-D67
Successful Make-up	$14.95	Phoenix, AZ 85048
Sports Recruiting:	$12.95	
Modeling:	$14.95	**Shipping:** $5.00 per book. Allow 7 days for delivery.
Wavy, Curly, Kinky	$14.95	**Sales Tax:** Add 7.05% to books shipped to Arizona addresses.
		Total enclosed: $_____

Printed in the United States
94624LV00001B/246/A